WITH THE BAND

How I Beat Overeating Through Lap-Band Surgery

VICTORIA ASHTON

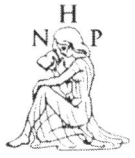

Northampton House Press

LIVING WITH THE BAND. Copyright 2013 by Victoria Ashton. All rights reserved, including the right to reproduce this book, or portions thereof, in any form.

Cover art by Naia Poyer from a photo by Robert Ander, by permission.

First Northampton House Press edition, 2013. ISBN 978-1482529-57-9.

10 9 8 7 6 5 4 3 2 1

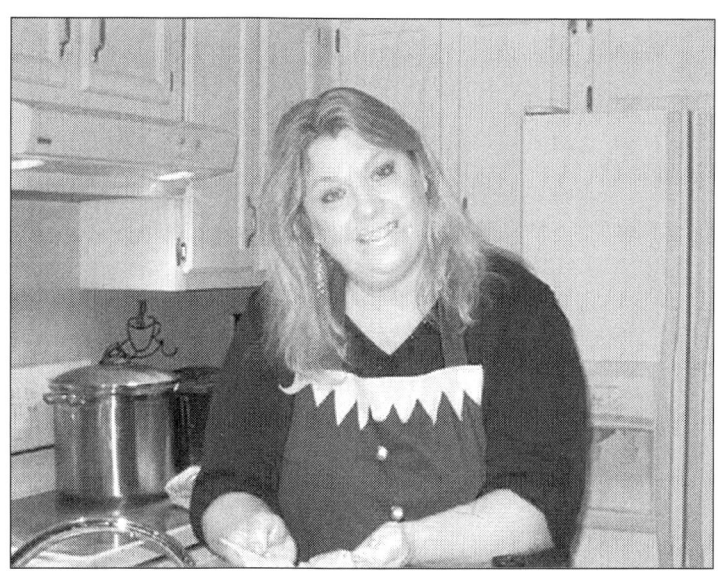

Victoria Ashton . . . *before*

VICTORIA ASHTON

LIVING WITH THE BAND

"I will never, ever get fat"

\- Victoria Ashton

INTRODUCTION AND PREFACE

    Morbid obesity is a serious disease, currently affecting more than six million Americans. It's associated with a number of life-threatening conditions, such as Type-2 diabetes, cancer, and hypertension, all of which can be improved with sufficient weight loss. Sometimes, when other methods have failed, surgery is the best option to use in taking control of your weight – and your life. Now an internationally-established procedure that eliminates many of the risks of other obesity surgeries is available in the United States. The LAP-BAND System is the only minimally invasive, adjustable and reversible FDA-approved surgical obesity treatment. It is an important tool which, properly used, can help improve your health, reduce your risk of developing associated severe medical conditions, and enhance the overall quality of your life.
    I know. This is the story of my experience with Lap-Band surgery, and beyond.

FOREWORD

by Dr. Mark Fontana, MD, FACS

Obesity is at epidemic proportions in the United States and has become a rapidly growing problem worldwide. 25 percent of all people in the industrialized world are now overweight. 17 percent of US children are obese and 35 percent of adults in the United States are now obese. In 2003, when I started performing this surgery as a major part of my clinical practice, surgery was beginning to be recognized as a powerful tool to combat the problem of obesity and improve or even cure many of the medical problems that can develop.

I didn't start my career as a bariatric surgeon. I trained as a physician and a surgeon through the US Navy and was stationed all over the world. In 2003 I went to war with the Marines and operated on US and Iraqi military personnel as well as Iraqi civilians. This was one of the most rewarding experiences of my life. I thought, at the time, that I would spend a career in the Navy with similar medical missions around the globe.

When I returned home, I was fortunate enough to spend a year with a partner and mentor, Dr. Jeff Lord, where I completed a year of laparoscopic and bariatric surgery training. We spent the year developing a state of the art program in weight loss surgery. It became evident that the military needed this care for dependents, spouses and military retirees. That was the year that changed the direction of my career and my life.

When I started down the road toward a career in "Advanced Laparoscopic Surgery", or surgery through multiple small (1/2 inch) incisions, I knew that I would like the technical aspects. It is cutting edge technology, difficult to perform, and the field was moving forward quickly with new techniques and devices. I never anticipated how much I would enjoy the patient care for this group of people. These were patients who'd decided to take a risk – to surgically change their bodies, implant devices, and learn again about eating, drinking and exercising to improve their health and wellbeing. There is nothing more professionally rewarding, than being entrusted by my patients to perform this surgery and participating in their unbelievable successes.

I left the Navy in 2005 and joined a growing bariatric practice in Norfolk, Virginia. My partner, Dr. Steve Wohlgemuth and I set out to make it the best program possible. Early on, the program our patients were required to complete was a cookbook of evaluations meant to select patients most likely to succeed, and education classes to give them the understanding and knowledge of how to utilize the surgical tool that they had chosen, whether it be the Lap Band, the gastric bypass or the sleeve gastrectomy. What I have found over the past 10 years and thousands of successful bariatric patients is that each patient is different with different needs. Where they come from, their personal baggage, their different abilities and their unique goals all combine to make each journey unique. I found that my initial emphasis on food choices, eating techniques and exercise goals was inadequate and far too simplistic an approach to give patients their best chance at success. An emphasis on expectations, psychological aspects of weight loss, body image changes and achieving happiness has found its way into our program.

There are a few patients in any surgeon's career who profoundly change how he or she practices medicine and surgery. Victoria is one of those patients. It was clear to me from the beginning that Victoria was determined to succeed and to change her life. She just needed the tool and to be pointed in the right direction and off she would go. She sailed through the education process and her surgery could not have gone any more smoothly. To say she was enthusiastic on the day of surgery would be a serious understatement!

It was only after surgery, when I would steer the office visits toward eating, drinking and exercise, and Victoria would steer right back to coping mechanisms, stress, family happiness and the control she achieved from her Lap Band, did I realize that she was showing me what she needed to help her with her journey. Many of the office visits had nothing to do with the use of the Lap Band but everything to do with her expectations, her new body image and the happiness with her success.

When my patients are successful for a year, I'm happy with them, but inform them that the journey is just beginning. Permanent changes in coping mechanisms, lifestyle and body image take time, and when a patient is successful for two years I am starting to see those changes take hold. Only when a patient has maintained weight loss, improved body image, managed expectations and fostered new coping mechanisms for the stresses of daily life, for 3 years, do I count him or her as a true success. It is by the third year that successful patients have faced their fear about weight regain, focused on themselves and what truly makes them happy – and at times, have had to leave doubters and enablers behind – that they know, deep inside, that they will never suffer from obesity again.

Victoria has passed her fourth year and continues her remarkable success. Success with weight loss, success with improved health, but most of all, happiness with the knowledge that her life has changed and she will not be going back to struggle with obesity again.

I hope you enjoy her journey as much as I have.

TABLE OF CONTENTS

Chapter 1. Fat Thighs	8
Chapter 2. My Unhappy Self	18
Chapter 3. Meet Doctor Fontana	26
Chapter 4. My New Path	32
Chapter 5. Hospital Hotel	38
Chapter 6. Darth Vader	42
Chapter 7. Your Surgery or Mine?	51
Chapter 8. Spread It Out	57
Chapter 9. I'm Starving	68
Chapter 10. I'm Not Alone	77
Chapter 11. Too Much Love	83
Chapter 12. Fourteen and Counting	88
Chapter 13. Hit Me with Your Best Shot	92
Chapter 14. The Last Straw	98
Chapter 15. Bad Breath Heaven	104
Chapter 16. Your Tool	109
Chapter 17. All Hands On Deck	114
Chapter 18. What Not To Do	119
Chapter 19. A Very Scary Evening	126
Chapter 20. Loose is Out	129
Chapter 21. Looking Back	138
Appendices:	
Victoria's List	142
Glossary of Terms	144

Chapter 1: Fat Thighs

By the time I was forty-seven, I no longer recognized the woman staring back at me from the mirror.

When I was a teenager, I used to look at women with big, heavy thighs and think how lucky I was my legs were stick thin. How could those women stand to have their fat rub together like that when they walked? Such thoughts started with me at a young age, and came naturally and frequently. So imagine my surprise when, a few decades later, I was looking in the mirror at thighs exactly like the ones I used to stare at in horror. Now every pair of jeans I owned ripped, the material getting thinner and thinner as my inner thighs rubbed with each step. I had become my own worst nightmare.

But wait - I was the pretty one! My father had said so. My sister, four years my senior, was the smart one. One off-hand comment, thrown out by my dominant parent, had determined the course of my life, which I had then lived unthinkingly. Until here I stood, staring in a full-length mirror, wondering what had gone wrong.

I'd always used my looks to get what I wanted. I'm not saying that proudly, but I was raised to believe women were supposed to do just that. My father had assured me my beauty would carry me through life; that the C's I received in school were adequate. Grades didn't matter, because I'd find a man to take care of me. And, well - he was right...sort of. I found many men, all willing to take care of me, in oh so many ways. Unfortunately they were all just like Dad: drowning in a sea of alcohol. My father, with each drink, had let his unhappiness float to the surface. Gradually he sank down, down, taking his family under with him. The men I dated, oddly, had all his familiar traits. Yet they still intrigued me enough that when they belittled and demeaned me, I would accept it, thinking in some sick way I must deserve it. Of course I can't totally put the blame on them. I steered the toboggan in my own downhill journey.

I spent my twenties traveling around the world as a flight attendant, kicking the nice guys to the curb. Then reveling in self-pity because of the abuse I suffered at the hands of the bad boys to whom I was attracted, over and over. I mistook swimming my way upstream through a churning sea of alcohol, screaming matches, verbal abuse, stomach aches, good sex, horrible sex, and even blacked out sex, for love, desire and devotion. Until, at the ripe old age of thirty-one, I finally met my match. My lover, a recovering alcoholic, beat the daylights out of me after giving in to booze again on our European vacation.

A talented DJ and musician, Andrew was used to getting female attention any time he craved it. But if I, his girlfriend, ever received any male come-ons, his jealously exploded. He'd punish me by not speaking for days at a time, leaving me devastated, and thinking I'd done something unforgivable. Finally, when he'd decided I'd suffered enough, he would beckon me over. Then, usually by requesting some sexual act, he would grudgingly let me back into his good graces. I got used to his silent treatment, and to all of his controlling comments. He would warn me to stay thin, literally directing my hand which held a bite of appetizer away from my mouth. I learned to avoid eye contact with male strangers, and to stay at home by myself when he was working. There were times when Andrew made me feel like the most beautiful woman in the world. But the truth is there were many more times when he made me feel stupid and ugly.

Our relationship gouged a thick scar on my heart and mind. I estranged myself from family because this man hungered to keep me all to himself. I was exhausted, thin, beaten down mentally and physically. But I never expected what happened one rainy, bleak night in Switzerland, far away from home.

We started our vacation in Paris with a drinking binge. Andrew had claimed sobriety for three years by then. With the exception of a capful of Nyquil taken to help fall asleep, I'd not seen alcohol pass his lips. But he'd just been let go from his job; his frustration was obvious. It was as if he'd forgotten all about his previous sobriety, and I could tell the job situation bothered him immensely. He angered easily. But now, instead of the silent treatment, he used all that pent-up energy to verbally abuse me. Soon, as we walked down the narrow streets of Paris, I was cringing any time a man looked my way. Andrew would always find some way to punish me for receiving attention I didn't ask for or even want.

As our vacation progressed and the days went on, his drinking worsened.

One night, after a long train ride to Switzerland, we sat in a dark bar not far from the station. I kept up as he ordered drink after drink. A couple was sitting across from us. Andrew stared at the woman's breasts spilling from her low-cut tank top, then muttered, "I betcha I could Frisbee this coaster from here and land it between those luscious beauties."

After years taking of abuse and torment from this man, and seeing him flirt (and no doubt later act on some of his uncouth suggestions) I simply cracked. All the alcohol I'd just chugged let me lower my guard long enough to reply, "Yeah, and I could probably French-kiss her boyfriend from here." I instantly regretted making the remark. Such crude commentary was his job, not mine. I could sense anger building as he snapped his fingers for the check.

The first blow struck me outside the bar. I didn't see his fist coming, and the punch knocked me off my feet and into the side of the building. Andrew then beat me as I tried to pull away; kicking and screaming as he dragged me all the way back to the hotel. I'd never experienced such strength and fury from one person. I felt totally helpless. People stared ... but nobody helped. Until at last someone pounded on our hotel room door, after he'd locked us in, an act which I believe literally saved my life. Only then did he stop hitting me.

The next morning, through one swollen black eye, I watched Andrew sob with his head in my lap, begging for forgiveness. *Déjà vu.* I had finally completed the transformation. I'd turned into my mother watching my father, in the same scene I'd witnessed in my youth so many times before. It was then, through the pitiful, hazy, morning-after fog that seemed to fill that tiny, cramped room, that something finally clicked in my brain. I'm not kidding: just like that. I knew suddenly that I was worth more than that ugly scene in the street. More than a headrest for some hung-over drunk sobbing insincerely in my lap. I was worth so much more than I was giving myself credit for.

But what was I going to do about it?

***

The time I spent licking my wounds in Europe after that terrifying escapade became the best three weeks I'd ever spent in bed. By then I'd worked up enough courage to be able to tell Andrew good-bye as soon as we landed back on US soil. Then, I immediately sought therapy. Now, at this point I could go on and on about my childhood, my insane choices of men, and the grueling depression that only lifted with a shot of Grand Marnier - but I think you probably already get the picture.

Sixteen days after leaving my abusive lover, I met Rick. At our first meeting, I considered him attractive enough, but about an hour into our conversation I suspected he still had unresolved feelings for an old girlfriend. She was the one who'd fixed us up. I had to wonder at her motives, a bit, too. So, I played therapist for a while, then hightailed it home. I didn't think twice about him, yet was not surprised to get a phone call two days later. After a few more dates, he assured me his feelings for his old flame were snuffed out. Although I was still focusing on picking myself up and dusting myself off from that last nightmare of a relationship, I was also beginning to enjoy my new friendship with this caring, uncomplicated man.

Rick, a true gentleman, was slowly growing on me. A nice guy wanted to take care of me. He acted as though he needed to take care of me. It would not have appealed to me before, but now . . .

Then, my phone rang at two o'clock one morning, and through the receiver I heard Andrew's sobs. He begged me to come back to him. I hung up, but knew I could forget sleep for the rest of the night. I turned the bath faucet on, hoping a long hot soak would help calm my nerves. I went down to the kitchen for a Diet Pepsi and was startled by the phone ringing once again. I made the mistake of answering and found myself listening to more of Andrew's smoldering self pity. Twenty minutes later I dragged myself back up the stairs and discovered a shallow river leading to the bathroom. I'd forgotten to turn off the faucet. I drained the water, laid towels all over the place, and went to bed. The next morning I packed my bag for my work trip, but when I walked downstairs I found part of my ceiling had fallen to the floor below after being soaked by the water.

The phone rang. This time it was Rick. Frantically I told him my story.

"Leave a key under your mat, Victoria," he said. "Go to work."

When I returned home, three days later, my ceiling was fixed, fresh flowers were in a vase on the table, and a card with a poem hand-written by Rick sat waiting for my arrival.

Of course if someone had told me back then I was going to marry this guy, I would've never believed them. If I'd met him six months earlier I would've considered him unchallenging. Too "nice!" Nowhere yet in my messed-up mind did I think of him as marriage material. But as my therapy (which he supported one hundred percent) progressed, for the first time in my adult life I felt loved in a way that I had never been before: with respect.

I knew this relationship was different. We were different. We took care of each other and slowly, calmly grew to love each other. I can't say it was easy or that our relationship always sailed on smooth waters. I bumped and bolted many times along the way, especially during our first year. But here is what I already knew by then: I wanted a partner; I wanted children; I wanted to never be yelled at and belittled again. I wanted my kids never to be yelled at. Yet I also didn't want the white picket fence. I knew with my creative, artsy-fartsy, acting, flying-and-fleeing background that I could paint that fence any color I wanted.
   We were married two and a half years after that first meeting. I was pregnant four months after the wedding. My life was getting better and better, and it was due to changes I had made. I was still a flight attendant, though.
    Back when I was twenty two, my acting teacher had told me, "Quit your flying job, Victoria. You'll get fat and lazy!"
   "No way!" I'd retorted. I love my flight schedule still. I like sleeping in on lazy mornings every week in different cities. I like the fast and unpredictable interaction with new people every time I go to work, and the money and benefits aren't anything to sneeze at, either. So my acting teacher had been only partially right.
   My father had been wrong, as well. By the time I was thirty-six, I actually had enough gumption to block out his misleading, twisted words. The ones that had left me always feeling pretty, but never

that I had enough intellect to study. With Rick's encouragement and my mother's and sisters' belief in my abilities, I earned a degree in psychology as I turned forty-two. My dad had died of cancer back when I was twenty-seven, so I was unable to brag to him about my academic accomplishment. What was more important was that I was proving it to myself. I'd married a Boy Scout whose love for me had been stronger than my own on our wedding day, but sometimes I wonder if I have him beat in that category today. We are raising two, beautiful, strong children, as a team. Together we make what the self-help books would call a wholesome, healthy family unit.

So how, you might wonder, was this acting teacher partly right?

I did get fat . . . and then fatter. Because depression followed, and food was comforting. So I got even fatter, and then I got sick. Sex, which had actually never been a strong point in our marriage, became nonexistent. What little self-esteem I had felt about my body went right out the window as those pounds kept packing on. As year after year went by I began to miss my old fun, misbehaving, co-dependent single friends. I missed being beautiful; being noticed. I missed the kind of wild, unmerciful sex I now saw only in movies. Basically, I missed all the old familiar chaos. I watched myself in the mirror growing older and heavier.

The only thing I felt grateful for was that I had my mother's skin. Soft, no stretch marks, no lines; in that category I was lucky. People still kept saying, "You don't look forty-seven!" But my oxygen level was sinking to seventy percent while I slept at night, depriving me of the normal ninety-eight percent your brain needs to function well and survive. I felt ninety-seven. I'd spent the last ten years in a sleepy fog, continuing to blossom and bloat.

Like every fat woman who berates herself before each shower, I'd tried every diet, program and pill on the market, before feeling despair and just giving in to flab. My husband and children were worried and wearied by my growing depression, but never once criticized my looks. No, I was my worst abuser. I pored over Dr. Phil's book on weight loss, and cried too - on many a night when I barely had enough energy to turn to the next page.

Then one day I received a phone call that would forever change my life, my health, and my soul. On the other end was one of my dearest friends, Joe, who had been very aware of my growing misery.

He said, "Victoria, have you ever heard of lap-band surgery?"

Chapter 2: My Unhappy Self

About a year earlier, I had watched an interesting television series about cosmetic surgery. I was intrigued every week by the petite doctor on the screen who deftly performed tummy tucks, face lifts, breast augmentation, and just about everything else that can be done to human flesh. Because my job allows me to fly anywhere in the country that my heart desires, I decided I wanted to meet her.

From the surgeon's T.V. show, I knew her office was in Los Angeles, so I made an appointment with her receptionist. I then took a working trip with a Los Angeles overnight. I had a twenty-four hour layover which I looked forward to with great excitement and even greater trepidation. I weighed about two-hundred and forty pounds at the time. Sweat poured off me as I thought about meeting this famous television doctor.

The cab ride seemed to take forever. Of course I had one of those drivers who took advantage of a captive audience to share her life story. It didn't really bother me, but I felt a little perturbed when she started hounding me to reveal mine. When I finally arrived and checked in, though, the doctor's staff put me at ease. I was relieved to find them quite friendly, despite the fame the show must have bestowed on the practice.

After a brief wait I was led back to a cubicle and instructed to undress to my underwear. The smell of sterile cleaning supplies filled my nostrils. I soon had one of those incredibly attractive, open-fronted, giant paper towels on, and was impatiently waiting for the doctor to enter. I sat stiffly upright on the cold metal table, trying to pretend my fat was not peeking out from the sides of my crisp, crackling, almost transparent robe. When she did finally come in, I noticed her protruding stomach and sincerely congratulated her on her second pregnancy.

She opened my robe and, like a housewife checking the quality of different cuts at the meat counter, nonchalantly started telling with me what could be done for my bloated body.

She pinched my large rounded midsection and said, "I could probably cut most of this off." Then she pinched both of my nipples and pulled and lifted them to the middle of my chest.

"They really should be up here," she said pulling and molding as if my breasts were mounds of meatloaf she was shaping for dinner.

"You would actually do better if you lost some weight first," she concluded. Then, as quickly as she'd come in, she was gone.

Lose some weight first? I was mortified. I dressed quickly, then grabbed another cab ride back to my hotel so I could sleep the rest of my time in Los Angeles away. After that blunt assessment, I felt as depressed as ever; destined to live the rest of my days as a fat woman.

Later that same year I made an appointment with a top cosmetic surgeon in my own area. Maybe, just maybe, I thought, this time the results will be different, and I can be helped.

Two residents watched him mark me up with a black sharpie. Then they took front and side-view pictures of my naked body. This doctor also mentioned I should lose weight before having any cosmetic surgery. I asked about a breast reduction, which I had convinced myself was my main goal since my shoulders and back ached from the two boulders I carried up front.

"Sure, I can do that," he said. "Then put implants in and make your breasts look perky."

I stared at him, my lower jaw nearly knocking the ground. I didn't want perky. For God's sake... I'd passed perky years ago! I just wanted less bulk, and maybe for my breasts to sit a little higher. I drove home feeling defeated again. No, feeling like an elephant in a side show.

Now here it was a year later, and I suddenly had high hopes about this lap-band surgery I was hearing all about from Joe, on the phone. This surgery might help me... it sounded as if it really could change my life!

***

Having children had also changed my life for the better. Except soon I'd have to stop using "having babies" as an excuse for weight gain, especially because they weren't babies anymore! I once asked my therapist why she thought I had gained so much weight over my married years.

"Well, Victoria," she said. "I honestly think it may be a way of protecting yourself. Using the fat to shield yourself from hurt, while discouraging outside male attention."

She had a point. I no longer could use my looks to get out of a speeding ticket, or get a free drink when I sidled up to a bar. Yet, I still didn't know how to feel; how to handle that. Married. I was *married.* With children. My life was theirs now. The question remained: What was left for me?

These days, my fat days, my two-hundred-and-forty-three-pound days, I didn't even want my own husband to want me anymore. Sex was too much work, and way too emotional. I didn't even like to touch my own body. I sure as hell didn't want anyone else touching it. I'd learned now what it felt like to be invisible. Men didn't pay attention to me anymore. Women didn't look at me with envy or dislike. More annoying, more mortifying, was that some of them seemed to look at me with sadness.

With some deep understanding that maybe a few of them held the secret to.

So what? I told myself. It's much easier to be invisible, to leave the flirting to the young...the attractive... those still willing to lie down. Now, I had more time to devote to my children, who did not lack for anything I could give them, within reason. I wanted them to be healthy and active. To follow every dream they could imagine.

All well and good. But also ironic, since I was not following *my* dreams. My health was fading fast. I did not eat healthy meals or snacks, nor could I expend any energy without becoming breathless. I barely made it through each day. I was great at giving my children the tools they needed for a healthy life. But I sucked at practicing what I preached.

My friend Joe seemed to know me better than I knew myself. On the phone he tuned into my misery and listened without interruption to my desire to find the real Victoria again. He had taken the time to research lap-band surgery. But after he told me all about it, and what the process involved, I told him I would never consider such a huge invasion of my body. Not that kind of critical adjustment made under the knife.

Ironically, here I was worried about a promising weight loss tool at a time when I could not make my body do any of the things it was supposed to do: Simple things, like walking up a flight of stairs without getting horribly winded. If I tried to run after a ball with my kids for more than a few minutes I would gasp and wheeze, feeling drained and ready for bed.

My children were worried about me. Mom never felt well. She was always tired. Mom just wasn't fun anymore.

My husband never complained, but I knew he missed the old me, too. He would talk of past vacations, when I used to swim and frolic (did I really just say frolic?) in the pool with him, as our kids swam around and around us, waiting for the perfect moment to launch a playful attack. He missed the Victoria he used to know – almost as much as I did. My entire family was concerned. As I got bigger and bigger, their fears grew larger and larger, the comments more pointed.

"You have such a pretty face."

"You would be so hot if you just lost some weight."

Man, oh man... *you have such a pretty face*. I hate *that* line in particular. It used to be what I'd mutter under my breath whenever I saw a bloated, overweight flight attendant adjusting her uniform, trying to tug it into place, while eating junk food between flights. Now I was that overweight, unhealthy woman in a too-tight uniform. The fat one I'd vowed I would never become.

Finally, with great humility, I accepted the information about lap-band surgery Joe had researched and labored over, and now held out to me with open arms.

What if? I thought. This just might work.

Thinking about it made me head right to Burger King, to ponder the situation as I consumed a double cheeseburger. I mean, if I was going to think of doing something that drastic, then I had better have my fill of junk food now. Am I right?

The biggest problem with that attitude was, when I craved this kind of fast-food crap, so did my children. My daughter and son often asked for greasy chicken nuggets and oily French fries. Why was I allowing all this saturated fat to flow into their little bodies and coat their brains? I was poisoning my own family, just as I had been poisoning myself for the past . . . how-many years? I'd lost track. And I was ashamed of myself.

When I was younger I'd never had the ability - no, that's the wrong word. I'd never had the stamina, will power, or desire to exercise properly – the right way. The healthy way. Back then, only one thing had helped my young, alcohol-saturated body stay in shape, and that was dancing. I could shake a leg with the best of them. Back then, I'd had two wonderful, platonic dancing partners and we'd spent many a night out until the dawn's early light. Oh lord, I'd had so much fun. Those were the days, my friend!

So where did that woman go? That fun-loving, beautiful woman I could no longer even catch a glimpse of reflected in an airport window as I walked by? An even more terrifying and surreal question was, what would I do with her if she resurfaced? I asked myself that over and over, and still wasn't sure of the answer. But I tell you what, by then I really wanted to find out!

My family and close friends all noticed a change in my mood. The problem had become a challenge, and I knew I'd have to show a lot of determination.

So, I made a list of the things I had to do in order to get the surgery I now craved and was focused on having, to improve my mental and physical health. I was ready to start checking those items off, one by one, and move myself closer to that goal.

Chapter 3: I Meet Doctor Fontana

It was late August, 2008 when my husband and I walked into the Heart Hospital for a lecture to be conducted by a bariatric surgeon on the facts about the lap-band procedure. I was stunned to see so many overweight people sitting in one room. Men and women - though mostly women - staring blankly ahead at the empty stage before them. I grabbed my husband's hand and pulled him up to two chairs front row and center. I wanted a complete, clear view of the thing that was about to change my life.

A model of a human stomach, pink and shaped like the letter S, loomed on the table in front of us. Suddenly I felt ready to bolt. The plastic stomach was squeezed at the top with a white plastic ring, which I assumed was the lap-band and not some giant, misplaced hair Scrunci. I gulped in my discomfort at seeing the possible future. My husband's skepticism and concern practically burned my arm as he leaned toward me protectively, instinctively.

After several more minutes of silent anticipation, a slight, middle aged woman rose and went up to the front to address the gathering. She was dressed in pale green scrubs, and spoke highly of the doctor we'd all come to hear. Her name was Jeanie, and she was Dr. Fontana's nurse. She started by explaining that she had gone through gastric bypass surgery three years before. I gotta tell ya... I was impressed. She looked good. She was energetic, she looked calm and seemed very healthy. All the things I longed to be. Slowly the tension left my shoulders. I glanced at the woman seated to my left, and smiled.

Dr. Fontana, an attractive man with dark hair and dark eyes, came in and took center stage after Jeanie's introduction. His immaculate white coat instantly gained my respect. All of us leaned a little forward in our seats to hear what he had to say.

He started by explaining gastric bypass and lap band surgery and what the differences were between them. "Two types of weight-loss surgery are the most common in the United States: gastric bypass and lap-band surgery. I'm going to talk a little bit about gastric bypass first."

We all looked up at the projected pictures on the pull-down screen: shining, rubbery-looking images of the human stomach. I felt a trickle of sweat creep down my spine. God, it was so foreign-looking. So icky and . . . alien.

"The gastric bypass is a restrictive procedure, which means that it limits the number of calories you can take in. That's because I actually cut, or divide, the upper stomach into a very small pouch. Now, if I left it divided like that the food would have no way of moving from the top of the stomach into the intestine, so I also cut the intestine and connect it to this new upper pouch. This procedure makes you feel full with a small meal, but some of the food goes right into the intestine and is not absorbed, because it's not been digested yet.

"So if you eat improperly, like sweets, you may get sick or feel nauseated. Good things, like vitamins and minerals, also take a little longer to be absorbed. So iron and calcium need to be taken in an extra high dose, like a supplement."

Okay. Wow. This sounded pleasant. I had already met people who'd had gastric bypass surgery, but hadn't known them well enough to ask about the intimate details. A friend's ex-wife had the procedure done and had lost over two hundred pounds. But he'd told me she also had anemia and a low-iron problem.

Sitting up straighter, I tried to shake the image of rerouted intestines out of my brain and concentrate, as Doctor Fontana continued with his testimony about lap-band surgery.

"The lap-band is restrictive and adjustable. What that means is, I place a small band around the top of the stomach. I don't need to cut the stomach or divide it. It's like a belt or band around the top.

On the inside of this band is a balloon that is adjustable."

I admit, the thought of a balloon simply resting on my stomach was a lot more appealing than having my intestines spliced and reconnected all over the place. But I still didn't know if all this seemed worth it yet. Doctor Fontana seemed so sure of himself, though. His confidence helped to put some of my doubts to rest.

"The band is attached to a small reservoir," he was saying now. "It's underneath the skin on the abdominal wall; nothing shows on the outside. When the patient is healed, I put a small needle into the port and inject saline solution or water into this band, which then squeezes the top of the stomach a little bit. It's adjustable, and restricts the amount you can eat because the food comes down and fills the small pouch. Food doesn't move through the band very quickly, so you feel satisfied with a small meal - as long as you're choosing the right food. Something liquid, like a milkshake, though, is going to go through very quickly. If it's steak, that'll take a while longer and make you feel full for a long time. So your food choices are very important with the lap-band."

I raised my hand. I had a ton of questions already, but one was weighing most heavily on my mind.

He looked at me. "Yes?"

"Are there a lot of complications with weight loss surgery?"

"The rate of complications for lap-band is about nine percent, meaning a little less than one out of ten people experience something we'd consider a complication. The most common are dehydration or nausea. Major problems are much lower than with gastric bypass, which has a complications rate of twenty-three percent."

Those statistics seemed comforting. The bottom line was, I had two children who deserved a healthy mother. I wanted to be able to keep up with them, not just watch them grow from the sidelines. I wished to be able to sleep well again. I craved the ability to simply walk up a few steps without panting. To feel good again, inside and out. Just listening to Dr. Fontana speak was making my heart palpitate and skip beats. My ill-spent past hadn't killed me, but I began to fear its results might; sooner rather than later.

After the meeting we all gathered around the front desk so Jeanie could measure our body mass index (BMI). I was stunned at what was actually considered 'obese'. I mean, yeah, I knew I was fat; but obese? And not just obese, but *morbidly* obese? That took me down a notch or two.

"Okay," I said to Dr. Fontana after that humbling experience. "I'm ready to go under. Where do I sign up?"

He stared at me blankly.

I thought, Oh boy. If this guy has no sense of humor, if he can't even see my distress well enough to understand it . . . well, I'm outta here.

Just then, he smiled.

Okay, I thought. *Okay.*

Chapter 4: My New Path

Doctor Fontana shook my hand as he entered the small examination room at Heart Hospital. This would be our first face-to-face meeting, and I must say I was nervous. A trickle of sweat traveled slowly down my spine and came to rest in a puddle near the top of my granny underwear.

"Looking at your chart, Victoria," he said, "I see you have a goal weight of one-hundred and fifty pounds. That's a healthy goal for your five-seven frame. Have you been taking our classes on the lap-band surgery and nutrition?"

I smiled triumphantly. "Yep. I'm on full speed ahead, even though I'm scared to death!"

"You'll do just fine," he answered. "Just remember the lap-band is a tool. Diet and exercise is the key to its success."

I felt relaxed in his presence. He didn't act rushed or disinterested like some doctors can seem - as if they view you more as an annoyance; merely an unfortunate interruption in their daily schedule. I felt reassured that I had the right team beside me, to guide me. Convinced Doctor Fontana was put in my path for a reason, and also convinced I was put into his for a reason.

    I was worried about all the testing to come, but also excited about finding out whether I had any health issues to be dealt with first, so I could, well . . . deal with them. Knowledge is power, and I was ready to take control. My day planner was filled with lap-band What To Do's and What Not To Do's, and my appointment book was filling up with each medical test or educational course I needed to complete. Once a week in the meetings I listened as people of all different shapes and sizes relayed personal stories of lap-band adventures. I was ready to embark on the journey that led to my own new path.

    All my life I've been greatly influenced by what other people think. Most of the decisions I've had to make, especially the important ones, I ran by close friends and family before I felt like I could continue. Knowing I had the approval of others has always motivated and given me a sense of purpose. Sometimes they offered positive insights; other times the feedback just reminded me of my lack of confidence. A slight sneer from Mom's lip, or the chiding click of Dad's tongue, could influence or even change a decision, even when I'd been totally confident of it just minutes before.

Well, this time my decision process was different. I was nervous but also defiant; more than ready for a fight when I told my friends and family that I was thinking of getting lap-band surgery. I learned one thing: everyone has an opinion. But this time, I decided I had to be selfish. I was in it for me.

My husband? No problem. He was with me all the way. He just wanted me to be happy again. "I love you the way you are, Victoria. So don't do this for me. Do this for yourself."

After being with so many men who had made up my mind for me on any life decision or cause I believed in, I can't tell you how refreshing Rick's attitude felt. One of the reasons I'd married him was because of his unwavering belief in me.

My mother? Hmmmph. My eighty-five-year-old mother who, to this day, can still run circles around me. Since my father died in 1986, she's blossomed into a confident, independent woman who lets no one tell her what to do.

"I'm going to church, then to the gym," she'll inform me on the phone. "Water aerobics. What're you doing today, Victoria? Why don't you take that silly dog of yours and go for a walk? Move your body. Why are you so tired?"

Many times she would look at me and shake her head. She just couldn't understand why I didn't just exercise and eat right. Well you know what? I didn't understand why not either! So how do you defend yourself in a case like that?

There's also my sister Marina. Eleven years my senior, born from my mother's first marriage. She definitely has genes my sister Valerie and I have only dreamed of possessing. Like my mother she exercises, eats the right way, and is determined and motivated to keep trim. A petite, fashion-oriented, get-up-and-work-out-at-five-A.M. type of gal. Good thing she's my sister, or I might hate her. She's disciplined with a capital D.

But me... when it came to exercise, I couldn't even manage discipline with a lower case d.

Then there's Valerie, my other sister, who was always dubbed "the smart one." My father's pet project. When I started talking about the lap-band, she had only two words for me. "DO IT!" she shouted.

"I've watched you get worse over the past few years, Victoria," she added, looking concerned and very serious. "The last time you came to visit it really scared me. Just walking seemed like a chore. I haven't seen you smile or laugh out loud in such a long time. I think you should go for it!"

But you know what? At this point I was already on full speed ahead, with a Do It or Die attitude. I was so sick and tired of being sick and tired that Oprah herself could've called and begged me not to have this surgery and I would've snubbed her. I was on a mission and damned if anyone or anything was going to stop me.

I couldn't remember the last time I hadn't felt tired all the time. Huffing up steps, lugging my suitcase like an anvil on overnight flights, feeling my legs shake and my heart race as I tried to catch my breath.

At my highest weight, two-hundred and forty-three pounds, I flew to London on a trans-Atlantic trip. I was so excited about finally being able to see the place my all-time favorite music idol, John Lennon, was from. This was one destination I'd saved up for a future adventure, and suddenly I was on my way.

Flying International felt quite different because I was so used to my domestic flight schedule. The extra long flights and change of time can mess you up for days. But here I was in my dream place! So when one of the other flight attendants offered to show me the ropes in London, I took advantage of her offer. En route to the city, another flight attendant saw us and joined our mission, which to my surprise pissed the first one off royally! Each woman literally each had me by one hand, dragging me along behind like a lost puppy, fighting over which place I should see first.

"I want to stop in this pub for a beer," one would say.

"No, no! There's a much cuter one down the block and across the street. Come on, Victoria."

"We need to get on the subway right here."

"Are you crazy? It's after dark... we need to walk. Come on, Victoria."

"I know a great place for dinner that serves the best fish and chips - "

"We don't want fish and chips. We want a nice juicy steak. Right, Victoria? Come on!"

It was not only mentally exhausting; physically it whipped my butt! Needless to say my saved-up, much-anticipated adventure was ultimately a flop. By the time I got back to the hotel room my legs felt like jelly. All I wanted was a cheeseburger and a soft place to land.

    So it was true. It'd been a very long time since I was able to keep up with people; I'd just given in and became a "slam-clicker" - an unsocial crew member who watched the world go by from her hotel room bed.

Now it was scary to have my body taken so seriously by everyone - friends, family, colleagues, medical professionals. Yet, at the same time, it felt quite comforting.

Was I as unhealthy on the inside as I was on the outside? I braced myself and waited to find out.

Chapter 5: Hospital Hotel

In the past, I'd never snored unless I was very tired- or very drunk. But these exhausting overweight days had made me a champion snorer without any help from outside influences. A serial dreamer, I would often wake myself with a loud snort. My husband, kids, sister, or whomever I happened to be napping around often mentioned how loudly I sawed logs in my sleep. I'd spent the last six years insisting to my primary care doctor, "My thyroid must be out of whack."

I wanted a test, or better yet, some medicine to fix it. There had to be a reason why I was walking through life in a hazy fog. Tired when I went to sleep, still tired when I woke. Tired when I ate, drank, peed, whatever. All the time just plain tired. Yet there seemed to be nothing I could do about it. At least, not till my friend Joe's phone call that night. Now perhaps I could look forward to a time when I'd once again wake up and feel rested. When I could go to bed and just quietly sleep.

Before a patient undergoes lap-band surgery, a large number of medical tests need to be performed. When Dr. Fontana's medical team interviewed me their first step was ordering a night in a sleep clinic for tests to see if they could identify just why I felt my brain was always in limbo. I was excited, nervous, and most of all *relieved*. Something was finally being done to look into my exhausted state and determine how to fix it.

On my appointment night, I walked the hospital halls looking unsuccessfully for the sleep apnea clinic. At last I was greeted in a stark-white hallway by a technician who asked, "Are you Victoria? I'm all set for you."

I was pleasantly surprised when she led me to a small room furnished and decorated to look exactly like a hotel room. *I've been a flight attendant for the last umpteen years,* I thought. *And stayed in every kind of hotel there is. This'll be a piece of cake!* It really didn't feel as if I was in a hospital at all. Double-sized bed, nice comfy recliner chair, a big television set. A large private bath and shower built into one corner. The whole set-up reeked of privacy and relaxation.

"Get your PJs on," said Maureen, my personal attendant. "Then brush your teeth and all that jazz, just like you're getting ready for bed at home. I'll call in over the speaker, and you can let me know when you're ready." She gave me a smile that made me feel I wasn't alone in this foreign adventure. Then she left me alone.

I pulled out silky tangerine-colored pajamas from Victoria's Secret that I'd bought five, maybe six years earlier. To my horror they barely buttoned. Jeez, these used to be big on me, I thought. Well, I *could* at least close the front. If not, wouldn't that have been just dandy! *Uh, excuse me? I gotta go home now; I can't fit into the pajamas I brought with me.*

Next I sat on a chair in a separate screening room, down the hall from my bedroom away from home, while Maureen glued tiny electrodes all over my head and body. Four televisions lit the screening room, each with a technician posted to supervise each patient who was being recorded in his or her own little hotel room just like mine. Yet totally unaware of all the snorting and sniffing, and God knows whatever other sounds they were all making.

I sat very still while the technician finished sticking at least twenty wired electrodes in total to my head, arms, legs and torso. All of them were connected to a machine that would record my actions and vital signs while I slept.

A half hour before, I'd gotten clearance to take an Ambien. I was beginning to feel drowsy as I walked back to my room, dragging all those skinny artificial octopus tentacles behind. I sat for a while and watched television in the comfortable lounge chair. Around eleven o'clock there came a strange whirrr. I looked up. A camera eyeball mounted at ceiling level was making its way around the room. It stopped right above me, staring down through its mechanical retina.

The voice of my attendant suddenly boomed over the speaker. "Okay, it's time to go to sleep now, Victoria."

I gave the eyeball a thumbs-up, then went to lie down on the nice double bed, wondering if I was actually going to be able to fall asleep. Impatiently I willed myself to relax; to ignore the insistent itching caused by the glue holding the electrodes in place. Finally, mercifully, the Ambien kicked in. Off to Never-Never Land I went.

I woke at five a.m. As my eyes fluttered open, I heard the same voice through the speakers on the wall. "We've recorded six hours already, Ms. Ashton. Would you like to leave earlier than six a.m.?"

Would I ever!

She came in and unplugged me. Fifteen minutes later I was back in my old minivan, on my way home.

Now, don't get me wrong. Nothing about the stay in the sleep clinic was painful. But it was a minor nuisance for some very little reasons. My long, hot shower at home felt so good. Even though I was still picking bits of sticky adhesive out of my hair days later. But what I found out next made it all worthwhile.

Chapter 6: Becoming Darth Vader

One week later the results were in. I walked into the doctor's office and anxiously stared into his eyes as he told me the sleep clinic results. I had mild sleep apnea, potentially a very dangerous condition. Life-threatening, in fact. A bariatric surgeon will not operate until you are successfully treated for it.

My pulmonary doctor suggested I try the C-Pap machine. "It's a device that opens your airway while you sleep, allowing you to breath with ease," he said.

After speaking with this specialist, I have to admit I was almost a little disappointed with the news. Mild sleep apnea alone still did not explain why I felt so horrible.

The nurse practitioner came into the room to explain in more detail how the C-pap machine works. We struck up a conversation, and I woefully told her of my lack of energy. My inability to sometimes make it through the day without longing to lie down.

"Sleep apnea could really cause me to feel this bad?" I asked. "I mean, there are times I simply cannot keep my eyes open. Sometimes I get twelve, thirteen, fourteen hours of sleep, yet still feel like I need another twelve, thirteen, fourteen hours."

"You know what, Victoria," she replied. "Let's try to test your oxygen level while you sleep. It wasn't bad when you did the test. Why not try it now and see what happens?"

She sent me home with a little machine the size of a kid's juice box, with a tube sticking out of it. You hook that up to one of your fingers like a clothes pin, and while you sleep it records oxygen levels.

I lay in bed wondering how I'd ever let my body get so far off track. For someone who had always put so much stock in her looks, I was still in shock at who I had gradually become.

"What the heck is that, Mom?" my son Dylan asked when he came in to say good-night. He pointed at the little box clipped to my index finger.

I explained what this little machine was there for, and saw the concern in his eyes. So I took his hand and gently clipped the clothespin device on his finger.

"See, Dylan? It doesn't hurt. I want to get better and have lots more energy. This is a good thing, sweetheart. I promise."

Two days later I was back in that same doctor's office, going over the results with the nurse-practitioner. She explained the readings she'd received from the box.

I was still puzzled. "So what does it mean that my oxygen level drops to seventy percent rather than stay around the normal ninety-eight percent?"

"Well," she began, "with that big a drop in oxygen to the brain, you could have a stroke or a heart attack. I'm sure that's why you're feeling so lethargic and depleted."

Bang, bang, bang went the trolley, ding, ding, ding, went the bell. Holy crap! No wonder I could barely move my tub-of-lard ass through my day.

I asked what I could do about it.

From that point on, out of my bedroom went the little bit of sensuality that was left. In moved a series of oxygen machines.

First I tried using the C-pap, a machine designed for sleep apnea patients. But I awoke at some point every night with my Darth Vader mask on the floor beside my bed, sucking up carpet pulp.

That machine was soon replaced with an oxygen tank that made my bedroom sound as if it had giant lungs pumping in and out all night long. The tank leaned like a wounded soldier in one corner of the bedroom, wheezing and groaning. Gradually I got used to snuffing up three litters of oxygen into my lungs, so they could send it up to my brain at night. It was going to make me feel better after all.

The first morning, though, after using my faithful tank all night, I felt like my head was going to explode. Suddenly I felt greater sympathy for people who have migraines! But gradually I got used to it. After three weeks the pulmonary doctor sent me home with that small box, again. The one that attaches to your finger while you sleep. It showed that by sleeping with the tank, my oxygen level was slowly creeping back into the normal category.

After about three months of this oxygen treatment, and feeling more energetic than I had in years, I paid a $495 dollar deposit to Dr. Fontana's office. The next process would be further testing on my all-but-broken body, moving me closer to the surgery that I was now longing to have.

***

When I began my treatment, the Heart Hospital in Virginia had a Bariatric Program Fee which included:

Pre-Surgical Nutritional and Exercise Education Session
Post-Surgical Nutritional and Exercise Education Session
Educational Material - Bariatric Program Patient Education Manual
RN Education, screening and coordination
Office visit co insurance/co pay, for visits prior to surgery
Free Weights
Pedometer

With payment of my fee, I also signed a letter of receipt, which read:

I understand that it is my responsibility to confirm Morbid Obesity Benefits for Bariatric Surgery (Lap Band/Gastric Bypass) with my insurance company prior to making this appointment. If it is determined by the surgeon on the day of my appointment that I am not a candidate for Bariatric surgery I will be refunded my program fee ($495.00) on that day.

I took my sleep clinic test results to a meeting with some of Dr. Fontana's staff. My pulmonary doctor had written to him, explaining that while I'd been unable to tolerate the C-Pap machine, he'd put me on three liters of oxygen and my level was now back to normal. I would have to continue treatment with the oxygen tank before and after my surgery.

At the office I met Lola, one of Doctor Fontana's assistants who handle insurance paperwork. It was there I discovered more of what is required for future candidates for the lap-band procedure.

Someone with a BMI of 40 or more;
Someone with diabetes or severe hypertension;
Someone with sleep apnea;

All are good candidates for their insurance to cover the surgery. Most insurance companies want documented doctor's proof of chronic obesity for the last seven years, as well as proof of failed diets such as Weight Watchers, Jenny Craig, or any other documented affiliations. Not a problem for me. I think I kept half of those programs open for the last ten years.

At our next meeting I asked Doctor Fontana why all of these classes and appointments were necessary. "Does everyone have to go through this complicated process? Are there any exceptions?"

"A multi-disciplinary team is very important, Victoria. We use a psychologist who knows how to deal with issues that can cause some people to gain or regain weight. An exercise physiologist, nutritionist, and other specialists are important links to a healthy recovery. The patients who continue to come back to those doctors for life-long reinforcement tend to keep the weight off."

I nodded. "I see. And I know my BMI is thirty-six. But I don't quite understand what that means."

"BMI is your body mass index which indicates how overweight you are," he explained. "A normal and healthy BMI would be 25. Surgery is beneficial with a BMI of over 35, when a patient has one of the three significant medical problems like diabetes, high blood pressure or sleep apnea. To know that is important, because the insurance companies follow this model. So if your biggest medical problem is arthritis, and your BMI is 37, the insurer is going to say that's not a life threatening medical problem. Then you aren't going to meet the criteria."

I nodded.

"If your BMI is over 40, you really don't need to have any other medical problems to qualify. But between 35 and 40, both insurance companies and doctors look for diabetes, high blood pressure, or sleep apnea, because we feel like treating those medical problems is very, very important. They also want to see documentation of other ways you've tried and failed to lose weight previously."

That made sense. If all noninvasive methods have failed, that clearly left surgery.

After my first office examination by Doctor Fontana, I made plans to attend the lap-band support group meetings and scheduled lab work, chest x-ray, EKG and clearance physician appointments and educational classes. Also, a psychological consultation and assessment is needed before surgery. I had to wait a couple of weeks for an appointment because all the recommended psychologists were quite busy. These specialized in the field of bariatric psychology. The ones I consulted really asked some eye-opening questions about depression, medications taken, past experiences with weight gain and weight loss.

I know this all must sound overwhelming. But I came to understand that it's a step by step process done for the patient's well being. My preparations and tests took about eight months to complete, but I've also heard of people finishing it all in just three short months.

At this point I worried I might not have the qualifications for my insurance company to agree to authorize the surgery. My BMI topped out at 36. I had no diabetes, no hypertension, and my sleep apnea was not really severe. Well, fine. I'd already made my decision. If necessary I'd take out a loan and pay for it all myself. Bye-bye to any new anything for awhile, but too bad. I just wanted to feel better. No - I needed to feel better.

At one point it did look as if I would have to dig deep into my own pocket to do so, though... but then came a miracle. I was approved! I guess when you can't breathe well enough to get proper oxygen, that is actually a little life threatening! Now it really was full steam ahead. I made plans. I made appointments I just could not get to fast enough!

Once again my friend Joe came through. He told me about a dentist in our area who specialized in sleep apnea patients. Suddenly I was looking at pictures of a dental night guard custom-made to fit my mouth; a small device which could possibly replace my oxygen machine at night. It's made from a mold of your teeth and when worn pulls the lower jaw out so your air passage remains open while you sleep.

I had one made for me, then tried to sleep while wearing it. It was a lot quieter than the hissing, wheezing Star Wars machine. Silent, in fact. Yet sure enough, many nights I would wake up and find that damned night guard lying like a dead mouse all the way across the room, just like the old Darth Vader mask.

Still, I did manage to do my finger-clip overnight sleep test with the new mouth guard planted firmly between my teeth, waking every so often to make sure it was still in place. Much to my delight, my oxygen level read as normal. Not only was that wonderful news, but the simple, silent device actually did stop my horrible snoring!

I still could not have my surgery until the sleep apnea issue was successfully addressed. At least I was able to get rid of that dreadful oxygen machine, as long as I slept with my night guard in. I did feel so much more rested when I woke with it in my mouth instead of swimming around in my bedcovers or buried behind a pillow or free-ranging across the carpet. I still sleep with my night guard in these days, and still cannot always keep it in my mouth all night long. After I told Doctor Fontana about the night guard, and how my oxygen levels were starting to come up to normal, he assured me that my time for surgery was near.

Chapter 7: Your Surgery or Mine?

It was January of 2008, just after my forty-seventh birthday. I sat in the Heart Hospital lobby waiting for the teacher of the lap-band class to arrive. Other people were waiting too, gripping the same white binder I held securely on my lap. The title, A Guide to Bariatric Surgery, seemed to glare at me from the front cover of the one held by a woman sitting on a couch directly across from me.

"Hi," I said to her. "When is your surgery?"

"March fifth," she replied, and gave me an uncertain smile.

I smiled back, and looked down at my book. *Lucky,* I thought. Seven whole days before mine. I just wanted this to be over with.

Jeanie, the same nurse I'd met at one of the support meetings, raced into the lobby with clipboard and pencil in hand. She greeted each person attached to a binder, then smiled and recorded names.

"And you are –?" she asked, looking down at me.

I was all but glued to the couch in anticipation. I couldn't believe I was really going through with this. "Hi Jeanie," I said.

She looked surprised when I said her name.

"I met you at a support group," I added. "I'm Victoria Ashton, the Diet Pepsi-aholic."

She laughed then. "And how's that going, Victoria?"

"I'm drinking as many as I can, as fast as I can, before my surgery." I grinned.

"Wrong answer." She laughed again, then flipped to the page for March twelfth on her clipboard, and put a check mark next to my name, just one more on a list of hopefuls. Turning back to me, she said, "You know, after my gastric bypass surgery I didn't have a soda for three and a half years. Then one day I took a sip of my friend's Diet Dr. Pepper and the cravings started all over again."

She turned away and headed across the room to the next patient.

What? I thought. What did she just say? I can't believe it. She'd sure sung a different tune at the lap-band support group, when I'd voiced my biggest fear, directing my comments right to Jeanie.

"I'm not scared of giving up any of the food, candy, or drinks at all," I'd said back then. "I'm only sad about giving up my one real addiction, Diet Pepsi." I'd felt actual caffeine tears filling the corners of my eyes.

See, with lap-band and with gastric bypass surgery, it's recommended that you give up all carbonated beverages. They can cause the digestive tract to bloat, and really make you feel horrible, as gas from the carbonation stretches your golf-ball-sized stomach. Yet, even knowing this, I still couldn't imagine being without the drink I'd been addicted to for the last thirty years of my life.

Jeanie, at that earlier support group, looked at me with such sympathy, then had confidently said, "Don't even worry another minute about that, Victoria. We'll help you with the cravings so it won't be a problem at all. We'll teach you what to drink and you won't think twice about giving up your Diet Pepsi."

Yet here she was, in the flesh, obviously not remembering those magic words that I'd hung on to for dear life. Now she was telling me she still craves Diet Dr. Pepper. I looked around in disbelief. *Okay, should I run now? I see the door, and my green, decrepit van peering at me from the parking lot. Maybe if I just...*

"Follow me, everyone," Jeanie said just then, foiling my plan for The Great Escape. She walked off at a pace that made me forget all about it, as we all trotted fast just to keep up.

Once inside the room she led us to, we each took one of the seats that surrounded a big U-shaped conference table. There were not that many, since each chair was about twice the size of a regular one.

"Hmm, my fat ass fits so well in this seat. I'm not hanging over the edge," the woman next to me said. She giggled and punched my arm playfully, but so hard it stung a bit. That was when I actually took a good look around and noticed I was the thinnest person, besides Jeanie, in the whole room. Usually I'd be looking around a room to see if I was the fattest, so this was a rare treat. Feeling thinner already, I settled on my oversized chair and opened my binder to the page Jeanie was instructing us to look at.

"By now," she began, "you all should be purchasing your liquids for the week before your surgery."

We all looked at each other like famished deer caught in ice-cream-truck head lights. This had to be by far the scariest way to begin. One whole week on nothing but liquids before having the surgery... seven whole days....seven! *Seite!* One, two, three, four, five, six, SEVEN!

After a moment we all smiled and nodded. *Yep, we're ready.*

Ready for a double cheeseburger from Burger King, my heart was really saying.

I'd spoken to a couple of women who'd already had the surgery. They gave me little tips on how to survive that long, lonely seven days. It was important not to cheat, I knew by then, because the fast helps your liver shrink a bit. Then your surgeon can manipulate around it better and have clear access to your stomach.

"I took a can of Campbell's cream of potato soup and strained it, then had that every night at dinner time," one woman had told me. "It seemed to help fill me up a bit."

I can handle that, I'd thought, back then. But now my emotions were beginning to take over. What if I couldn't handle it? *If I give up my comfort food, what will I have left?*

"Remember," continued Jeanie, "Twenty grams of protein a day for that week only. You can have sugar-free yogurt."

Great. I hate yogurt.

"Oh, and sugar-free puddings."

I hate puddings even more.

"Plus skim milk."

Surprise! I hate all things milk.

"Of course beef or chicken broth is a great way to get in your protein every day."

Of course it is. I've never been able to stand sipping plain chicken broth or beef broth.

I raised my hand.

"Yes, Victoria?"

"Can I have wonton soup broth?" I asked, holding my breath.

"Yes, sure you can. Just the broth."

Phew, I thought, saved again. I do love wonton soup.

The room grew quiet as we all started bundling up our papers for the journey home.

"Good luck everybody," Jeanie said, in a slightly high, sing-song kind of voice. "And don't cheat!"

I drove slowly, thinking of the process that lay ahead. I stopped at the grocery store and purchased about ten cans of Campbell's cream of potato soup. Back in the car my brain would not stop chanting...*no more fast food, no more Diet Pepsi, no more potato chips and onion dip....*

Wait. No more potato chips and onion dip, *ever?* My fasting days had not yet begun. I turned my van around and drove back to the store.

Chapter 8: Spread It Out

Up to the time I decided to have my surgery, my life philosophy had been: *If I had to get fat at least when I did gain weight it went everywhere, not just to one place.*

And it's true. I had gained all over. I didn't have enormous hips, or a butt the size of Texas; I'd spread out equally. Thank the Lord for little miracles. So if I dressed carefully, with attention to slimming colors and combinations, most people never guessed I weighed as much as I did. But if they'd ever seen me naked-a thing which I couldn't even bear to think about – then they would've known in an instant.

But I'd become pretty talented at camouflaging the weight by keeping my entire closet stocked with black and grey clothing. In the summertime I suffered and sweated in long-sleeved black shirts layered under what I'd convinced myself were attractively slimming jackets. At work other flight attendants and pilots used to make comments about all of the layers I had on. If I saw someone in the crew lounge who'd known me for many years, and I hadn't seen them in a long time, I would actually hide rather than face them and the inevitable look of surprise. I was mortified by my appearance. In fact, I could not stand to even look at myself. I carefully avoided mirrors, especially full-length ones.

When I worked I carried a battery-operated fan that also squirted a fine mist of water, because I was constantly sweating. I wasn't sure if I was experiencing hot flashes – you know, that wonderful endless peri-menopausal stage when a woman feels like she's being teleported back and forth between a tropical forest and the real landscape, where everyone else feels fine or is even shivering? Or if it was the layer upon layer of concealing clothing that was getting to me. Probably both, come to think of it.

It is so exhausting being fat!

Another thing I'd noticed: Airplane seats were getting smaller. I couldn't admit the problem was really me, getting bigger.

Just making through one of my normal flying trips was painful. I wasted so many overnights, if I had any amount of time in a place, taking a long bath to erase the accumulated sweat of the day. Then I'd slide beneath the sheets (no matter what time of day it was) and stay there until an hour before I was to meet the crew and depart. A 'slam-clicker' is what I was dubbed. As a younger flight attendant I'd explore each city after I arrived, taking in all the sights, catching a new play or a first-run movie. Or I'd have a nice dinner with the crew. By then I'd also learned how to be comfortable simply on my own, and had no qualms about also trying out new foods and exciting restaurants as a party of one.

But nowadays room service was my best friend. All by myself, in the hotel room, I could eat what I wanted without anyone seeing what I choose or how much I swallowed, and judging me. Potato skins and nachos were a staple meal. Even though I liked salads and chicken, they were never my first choice.

One thing for sure: It's very difficult to find healthy food choices at American airports. Once you start taking notice of what you eat, and how you eat, and how you must get those things to eat, and where you can buy them, it's definitely a wake-up call. Also an eye-opening commentary on why America has such a severe obesity problem.

Now, even back then I knew eating healthy was possible. I'd flown with plenty of flight attendants who lugged along their own food. Often several small blue coolers (to match their uniform bags) sat scattered about the crew room, as if mocking me. Or maybe just trying to show me the way it can be done. It's a lot of extra work to keep everything iced, and you need to know what you can prepare and where it can be done. But you know what? You have to decide you're worth it. And the money you save by not purchasing airport food and room service! Dang! Breakfast, lunch and dinner on a four-day trip can really rack it up.

    Heavy as I was back then, it seemed like I was always on a diet. "Yo-Yo Effect" was my middle name. Lose twenty pounds, gain back twenty-two. Go on a new fad diet and lose fifteen pounds, then gain seventeen back. Fasting, protein only, bags and bags of grapefruits, shredded cabbage... yada, yada, yada. Every year, on the first day of January, the same resolution: I will lose weight this year, and be thin again. Yet each last day of December I could've climbed on that dreaded bathroom scale and seen higher numbers.

    God, I was tired. Of all that, and of me. But now I was going to do something more effective than any fad diet. I was going to make a real change, not a temporary one.

    The days seemed to pass slowly as I waited for the surgery date to draw near. Wow, I thought. I can't believe I'm actually going through with this! It's really happening, and I'm the one making it happen. Look out world, Victoria is coming back to the land of the living.

    My son, in third grade at the time, came home from school one afternoon and told me one of his teachers had recently had lap-band surgery.

    "Mom," he began, "she went from being bigger than you to WOW!"

    That made me feel so good. No, not just good. It made me feel great, and so hopeful. I've noticed an amazing thing: When you hear of something new, or you are questioning some kind of procedure or big step, all of a sudden you run into other people on the same wavelength, who are also hoping to achieve the same fate. Karma, cosmic synchronicity, pure coincidence, whatever you what to call it – it really is amazing. All of a sudden it seemed I knew of six people who'd had or were thinking of having lap-band surgery. And the ones who'd already had it were doing quite well. So if they could do this and come away with such awesome results, why couldn't I?

    Still, from time to time I'd suffer sudden attacks of guilt. Why didn't I just have the damn willpower to lose all that weight? Was this merely a selfish endeavor, instead of a vital tool needed to save my life? But the more I read about the surgery, and the more I talked to people about it, the more I believed in and wanted it.

    I was scared to move forward, but even more scared not to. Doctor Fontana's group had warned me to be careful of what I ate in the days leading up to my surgery. They'd already weighed me in; that was the base number that they would be going by from now on. They made sure to remind me that if a patient gained twelve pounds or more, then going forward with the surgery on that date would no longer be an option. Those numbers, and that result, both felt like they'd been seared like a USDA brand in my brain.

    Intellectually I really wanted to do everything they told me; eat correctly, lose weight, start weaning myself off the divine nectar of the gods also known as Diet Pepsi. Yet somehow my stomach was still on automatic pilot. Burger King, Chinese food, Dairy Queen – which oddly enough I had only started craving after my decision to go for the surgery. And Taco Bell, of course, my favorite. I was running on pure addiction; on carbs and fat and adrenaline. But I felt like I couldn't help it, and convinced myself each time, "This bad meal is close to being my last!"

Here's a perfect example. I was on a flight trip with a male attendant who'd had the surgery done six months before I'd met him. "I can have one piece of pizza," he explained. "But if I have two? Then I lose it." Meaning, he would throw up.

I felt as if I'd just witnessed the climactic scene in a horror movie.

So what did I then proceed to do? That night on the overnight I ordered a fourteen-inch pizza and made damn sure I ate as much of it as I could. After all, I told myself, this just might be my last pizza ever in the world. Of course I knew this behavior was dangerous, and that my eating was out of control. I was not handling this process correctly – and certainly not letting anyone even closer to me than that flight attendant know about it.

Because, maybe if no one knew then it wasn't really so bad. Maybe if nobody found out, then it wasn't even real!

I still had a deep fear of letting people down, even though when I did usually it was really me I'd ended up disappointing. That's why I'd developed a pattern of quitting projects or giving up on goals when I was halfway there. I'd get overwhelmed and insecure. I still have half-written books in every drawer of my room. Not to mention other creative endeavors I'd started, then left to fizzle. Because I'd already flitted on to the next project, leaving all thoughts of the previous one behind. Lap-band surgery was the road to reaching the biggest want and desire I'd ever taken on in my life. I really wasn't doing this for anyone else. I was doing it for me this time, and positive I was making the right decision. Why? Because I wanted to enjoy my children before they were all grown up and had moved away from my nest. I wanted to participate in their lives, not just sit like a lump on the sidelines, out of breath, and watch them zip by. I also did not want to see the kids turn into another version of me. That old 'Do as I Say, Not as I Do' attitude that I still had was simply not cutting it anymore. I was an unhealthy, overweight, lethargic, no-clothes-that-fit-me kind of woman. Still growing out, not up; getting bigger and bigger and bigger. I understood finally time was running out... and I could not believe how many years I had already wasted.

Experts say people waste a certain amount of their lives standing in lines. I began to wonder how much of our lives fat people wasted lying in bed.

Actually, I had a pretty good idea. On the job I was not able to take the real hard-working trips because I just could not make it through that sort of day anymore without being exhausted. Sometimes I'd serve a flight, then go to the airplane bathroom and rest my head on the little metal sink, trying to find enough energy to make it through the rest of the flight. At the end of the day I'd almost burst into tears when we landed. Not from feeling I'd been in any danger, but rather from relief. From knowing soon I'd be lying in bed watching TV and relaxing.

I could've gotten clinically depressed about my fat self very easily. If I were not a stronger person, or did not have my children to think of, it would've been very easy to climb into bed and simply not get up again. The sad truth is, by then I hated myself. I hated my body. When I did force myself to dress and go out somewhere, it was like being sent down to Hell. Always feeling the trickle of sweat under the cups of my bra, as it slowly made its way down to soak into my girdle.

At my brother-in-law's wedding, five years earlier, I'd had an unusual burst of energy. That night I was really enjoy dancing with all of the kids and my husband at the reception; I actually was doing some old dance moves, feeling unusually happy and energized. After an hour or so, I slipped into the bathroom for the demeaning task of unclipping this set of hooks, pulling off that elastic, unzipping whatever was holding me in, simply so I could use the restroom.

Once inside I glanced in the mirror and froze in horror. My face was beet red, my hair sopping wet from all the sweat I'd generated dancing. After recovering from the horrible sight staring back from the mirror, I tidied up to make myself more presentable. Then I sat out the rest of the night. And it saddened me terribly.

Back in my twenties, if I gained any weight I could starve myself for a couple of days and be right back to my shining, thin old self. But now my fat self could starve for weeks and end up just gaining more weight. It was exhausting, and no way to live.

I'd gained a lot of weight when I went back to college at forty. I took a leave of absence from flying and attended Virginia Wesleyan to earn my bachelor's degree in psychology. Suddenly I found myself surrounded by younger students, a totally different scene than when I'd gotten my Associates degree by going to night school at Tidewater Community College three years before. There I'd blended in with the other older, wannabe graduates. I'd made some friends. But every day at Wesleyan I was separate, camouflaged in sweatpants and loose T-shirts. I never felt I belonged.

When I went back to flying a year and a half later, none of my uniforms fit anymore. I was mortified. The first time I dressed to go back to work, my bodysuit stuck as I tried to pull it down and then back up over my chest. It was lodged like a big rubber band around my midsection. I made a joke about it on the outside, but on the inside I was dying. We all go through so much just trying to hold our fat in. Stuff it in that bodysuit, plunge it through that elastic hole. We are what we are. But it's up to us to change ourselves or quit bitching about our lives in the process.

This was my new attitude: Come hell or high water, I was ready. Nothing would be put away in a drawer to be forgotten. Not this time.

My son was scared, though, and he said so. "What if they put you to sleep and you don't wake up?" he asked me more than once. He's a boy who's not afraid to tell you exactly what he's feeling, one of the qualities I love and admire about him most. He kept on telling me, "You're not fat, Mom. I love you just the way you are."

I tried to explain that I didn't love me the way I was, so I needed to make myself better. If I wanted to see him grow up, I needed to change and become healthy. Then I could be around for his children, too, one day.

My daughter's different. She always suffers in silence. That worries me so much it just about kills me every day. I knew she was scared about the upcoming surgery. I could feel fear seeping out of her every pore. I didn't like to just smile and say, "Mom's going to be fine" because I didn't know that for sure. But I did tell her I was doing my best to change and be healthy – not just for myself but for her and her brother. She manifests stress so differently than my son; a lot like me, actually. She gets stomachaches and headaches, then withdrawals quietly into herself. She's very creative, thank goodness. She can spend hour after hour releasing pictures from her left hand onto a fresh piece of clean, unlined paper – and in this way lifting her mind free of a burden.

I did know both kids would support me, and that was more than I could ask for. I was worried about worrying them, but just kept telling myself: Soon they're going to have a healthy mother.

I was hoping and praying this surgery would change all our lives.

Then, in a meeting in early February with Doctor Fontana, I learned I had blossomed from 239 to 243 pounds. Who the hell was this sick chick? Why couldn't I get her under control? The more I thought about it, the more emotional I got. The more upset I got, the more I ate. I was disappointing myself, and now it felt like I was disappointing my doctor as well. I felt like a failure, ready to throw in the towel even before the real journey began.

Then I met a young woman in the waiting room. We stuck up a conversation. She was scheduled to have her surgery five days before I was supposed to have mine.

"I gained four pounds," I said. I'm sure the disappointment and self-loathing showed on my face.

"Don't feel bad," she answered. "I wish I'd only gained four pounds. I gained twelve."

Wow. I thought. Oh, wow.

I left that office a little later with a bounce in my step. Maybe I wasn't doing as badly as I thought. And the greatest thing was, I drove right past every fast food place on the way home.

Chapter 9: I Think I'm Starving!

Okay, now for the really fun part: the week of the fast. After I'd sat and looked around at everyone's faces, at the stunned expressions as our nutritionist explained what it was we could (but mostly could not) eat, I went right out to a health food and vitamin store and bought one of each product she'd recommended. Protein shakes, clear liquids, tubes of this, tubes of that. I didn't sample all of them, like I'd said I would. But I bought plenty of samples to taste before buying so I'd have a better idea of what I could tolerate. And the first day of my fast I did just fine.

Of course, what I haven't told you is how I had to hold my nose as I sucked down those thick, slimy liquids. They reminded me of the Slim-fast diet. I know there are people who like the taste of those vitamin drinks – my husband and mother included. Folks who would readily substitute one of these flavored canned liquids for a real meal some days. Not me. The second day by lunch time I was so hungry I went to a Chinese restaurant and stocked up on take-out cartons of wonton soup without the wontons. Yep, you heard me right... "Wonton soup, please hold the wontons." Yummy. Hot and filling – and clear. Yet it tasted like real food!

I must say, by the third day (by which time I'd been told the strong hunger feeling was supposed to ease, and the fast get easier,) I was absolutely starving.

So now I'm going to confess something I did which I have not yet told another soul, until now: I cheated. I went to Burger King and got a huge, and I mean huge, double cheeseburger. I finished it before I hit the first stop light on the way home. While sitting at the next light I looked over at a Taco Bell across the street and heard it calling my name. I have never longed for food so desperately. Forbidden! Off limits! No, no, no. Well? What could it hurt? I'd already blown the liquid diet, big time. And so, just like with all my previous "I'll start over tomorrow diets," I turned into the drive-through there, as well, and got myself two crunchy hard tacos.

After eating them, I felt so disgusted with myself, I cried all the way home.

By this time I was also supposed to have limited contact with my love-hate nemesis Diet Pepsi to a minimum. Yet I was still drinking a ton of those even as I was going through a grieving process about their impending demise. It felt like I was saying good-bye to a dear friend; one whom I did not know if I would ever see again. Emotional, gotta tell ya. Very emotional.

"Victoria, aren't you supposed to limit your Diet Pepsi intake?" Joe asked me once, when I ordered an extra-large soda after sweating all morning on one of our yard-sale jaunts.

"I am!" I fired back defensively. "This is the first one in two days," I lied.

His disapproving look showed me I was not fooling anyone, not even myself. Any time I allowed a setback like that, it only made it that much harder to resist more temptations. I felt alone, frustrated, afraid. Here I'd told everyone what I was doing, and now I was already failing.

I decided to try harder.

I simply could not stand the protein shakes. The dread and repulsion they aroused in me were one reason I was having such a hard time adhering to the fast. Instead I stuck with vitamins, wonton broth, and then – on the advice of a fellow "lap-bander" – I lapped up Campbell's low-sodium Cream of Potato Soup, making sure to strain all of the potatoes out before I ate it. A little pepper on that, and I was good to go. This addition to the diet was immensely helpful. So much so that I did not cheat again with my old stand-by fast food places. I had a couple handfuls of raw vegetables, and on day six one-half of a grilled chicken breast. But is that really cheating if it's healthy and keeps you honest the rest of the time? I kept telling myself, "It's only for seven days." And, "You can do this." I was still anxious to change my life and health for the better, and really did not want to screw everything up.

I made it through the whole seven days without feeling like a complete failure. I must say, I was even a little proud of myself. I didn't weigh myself even once during that week because I was worried that if I didn't see any loss, I'd really freak and go out and eat a whole cow. I was trying hard to stay in the right mind set. Thank goodness for Doctor Fontana, his staff, and my family. In the end I had all the support around me that I needed.

And please, please, please understand this: plenty of choices were given to me on what I could safely eat for this fast. I'm making jokes now about certain aspects of that experience, but I strongly recommend you take this part very seriously and listen to your nutritionist. In retrospect, obviously I don't feel like I did it in the most correct manner. Instead I did what I had to do, to get by. I knew in the end what would work for me. In any case, I did do exactly what I try to also teach my children, every day, which is "Just do your best." Many other options, such as yogurts, protein bars, protein shakes, and puddings were offered to me as well. I rejected these because I am such a picky eater and dairy-phobe. Unfortunately, I'm even more picky when it comes to healthy foods than I am with junk! We all know what a steady diet of that will do for you.

Yes, there were some vegetables I liked, and some fruits. Many of these I hadn't even tasted in years. I am definitely a confirmed carnivore. Steak, chicken, and pork are my staples. Fish? Unfortunately, I hate seafood. All seafood! Oh, I know what you're saying to yourself right now. "Well she hasn't tried my shrimp or my fish – not the special way I prepare it." Or, "When I make swordfish it tastes just like chicken." I hate that line, and I've heard them all. My answer: Why would I even want to taste something that "tastes just like chicken," but isn't? I'll just eat chicken, thank you very much!

So here I am, not a healthy eater – in fact, a very *picky* unhealthy eater. And now all the foods I loved and craved most – potatoes, breads, pastas – were all going on a taboo list. Holy crap, I was scared. Terrified, in fact. My family watched me go through this week with bated breath, waiting to see what would happen. I made sure I did not go into the kitchen and or do any cooking for the entire length of the fast. Instead, the week before, I'd frozen for my family a pan of lasagna and a shepherd's pie. While they were eating these I'd run errands or go take a long hot soak in my bathtub, with the door shut against any tempting smells. I also pouted a lot, I'm not proud to confess, wondering if I'd even made the right decision. Many, many times doubts filled my mind, as I asked myself variations of that question over and over again.

But I would not know what I weighed until the actual day of surgery. So I did not step on any scale, for fear of being my own major disappointment.

One night before the surgery, I was in a music studio working on a song an old friend and I had written. The man who owned the studio had known me back when I was seventeen; he hadn't seen me a whole heck of a lot through the years. When he walked into the studio he looked at me and exclaimed, "Oh, man, Victoria...you've gotten so fat!"

I was devastated, and literally speechless. That insensitive remark felt like a physical burn all over my skin. I couldn't think of anything else for the rest of the night. The glory I should've felt about my song being born that night had been tainted. Once again I found myself crying all the way home. When I got there, my worried friend – the one I'd partnered with on the song – called me up to see if I was okay.

"Don't pay attention him, Victoria," he said. "The man doesn't ever think before he speaks."

"But – do you think I'm fat?" I asked between sobs.

"The truth is in the mirror," he said. "You have to decide. I'd still love you whether you were one hundred twenty pounds or three hundred twenty."

That was nice to hear from someone who had also known the skinny me. But I knew the truth. I was fat, and I absolutely hated it.

That incident made me think hard, though. I am definitely a people pleaser and there are certain people I've always wanted to make happy. It wasn't until recently, after all the work I'd been doing with the lap-band, that I came to realize something life-changing: *The only really important influence on your image is acceptance of yourself.*

So, if you are overweight, but comfortable and happy, and you don't care about others' opinions, then good for you. Don't change, unless it's necessary for health reasons. But me? I hadn't been happy in my own body for years. I knew I had to do something drastic, and soon, because I was going under, emotionally and physically. Getting fatter and fatter, sicker and sicker. And yet I'd never even been to the hospital before, for any kind of surgery, except an outpatient procedure on my cervix. An experience that was in a league all by itself.

Let me pause here to stress the importance of regular yearly check-ups.

Three years before my lap-band experience I went to my gynecologist for a regular, scheduled pap smear. I'm like clockwork every year for that exam, and always had normal results. But this time, a week after being seen by my doctor, I got a phone call from a nurse on her staff, who said I'd had an abnormal pap-smear result.

Hmmmm, I thought. Okay. I'd heard stories of lab work being messed up; maybe mine had just been one of those. When I got to the office, my very southern doctor said "Vicky." God, yes – she calls me Vicky. "Yoah pap smear is just not abnahhmal, its showing that you have seveah dysplasia."

I think I just stared. "What?" Because I already knew that dysplasia comes in stages – one through four. So why and how did I go from "normal" in the last exam to severe (the next step away from cancer) all in one year?

"Ah need to do a biopsy on you, Vicky. So take the bottom part of all yoah clothes off and get up on the table. Ah'll be back in a few." Then she left.

Well, I lay on the cold steel table, trying to keep covered under the midget blanket, heart pounding like a shoemaker's hammer. Fear crept in trickles of ice water through every part of body and soul. What if I had cancer? God, I was scared.

Then all of a sudden, I heard it. *Beep-beep-beep-beep-beep-beep.*

"What the hell?" I muttered. *Beep-beep-beep.* It was the freaking fire alarm. "You have got to be kidding me," I said to the ceiling.

My doctor flew back into the examining room. "Vicky, put yoah pants on. We need to go outside!"

Unbelievable. As I trekked down the four flights of stairs I felt like running away. My doctor stayed right by my side until it was time to go back in. I think she could sense my fight-or-flight reaction.

The next thing I knew I was back on the table. The biopsy definitely was a bit uncomfortable. But, mercifully, it was over before I had a chance to say "I'm getting the hell out of here!"

My results came in the following week. They confirmed I had severe dysplasia of the cervix. From there everything happened very fast. I was scheduled for a LEEP procedure immediately. My doctor described, in her signature thick southern drawl, what she would be doing to me. "It'll be lahk takin' a hot knife and slicin' through buttah." She would cut away the diseased layers of my cervix and we'd hope that would do the trick.

That surgery was uneventful. I needed to go back in every three months for a follow-up. And man, did she follow-up, and up. Then it was only every six months. Now I'm back to my regular, once-a-year check up. Today I'm also back to having normal pap tests, because a potentially-fatal disease was caught in time. So ladies, listen to me. One of the reasons I'm telling this story is to beg and plead: When you're thinking of your health, be sure to also get your pap smear done once a year. Things can change in an instant. Your life may depend on knowing that they have!

Anyways, that LEEP was the only surgical procedure I'd ever had done before suddenly finding myself lying on a hospital gurney, being prepped and wheeled in for the lap-band procedure. But I felt safe with Doctor Fontana, just as I'd felt safe with my gynecologist. That's why it's so important to have a good relationship with doctors, and feel you trust yours. *If you don't, find another one immediately.*

Chapter 10: I'm Not Alone

Lying on that gurney, thinking back over the past eight months while all that lap-band testing was being accomplished, I felt amazed at how far I'd come. Some of the final tests had just been exciting; some quite nerve-racking. And some, well – downright scary.

The night before surgery I was kind of on automatic pilot. Get dinner on time for the kids, clean out the kitty litter, answer the phone call from my mother, clean up the kitchen, answer another call from my mother . . . you know, the usual. I felt like I ought to keep busy. I had to keep my pair of "You're Foolish" and "You're Selfish" demons at bay.

So naturally I thank the good Lord to have been blessed with an irreplaceable, wonderful best friend. Sex and the City girlfriends have nothing on us. Over the past twenty years Jody and I have been through more ups and downs, more zigs and zags, more tit for tat, than any two friends should have to take. Abusive boyfriends, wayward friends, marriage, miscarriage, premature birth, gay spouse, divorce, pushy parents, therapy. You name it, and one or even both of us have been through it. The single constant in our lives has always been each other. Jody was totally supportive of my lap-band decision. She flew in from Ohio, leaving her two young daughters with her sister, so she could be by my side. I cannot express what this meant to me. I wouldn't hesitate to be by her side, or anyone else's for that matter. But I've never been comfortable with accepting reciprocation from others. Yet on this night I could not have been more grateful to have her there with me.

Sleep did not come easy. But by five the next morning Jody, my husband Rick and I were on the highway heading towards the surgical start of my new life. On the surface I think I looked as if I had nerves of steel. But on the inside, just like Meryl Streep in that movie "The Bridges of Madison County", one hand was on the door handle. Jump out! Run, run, run for your life! I thought. Just as I had wished for Francesca/Meryl to jump out of that damned truck and back into Clint's arms. I mean, Clint Eastwood, for God's sake!

Anyways, I sat quite still, listening to my husband's nervous whistling, wondering if this might be my last morning on earth. I'd never been put under before, unless you count that stuff they dose you with for a colonoscopy. I'm not sure what drug it was they gave me for that procedure, another test you must endure before having lap-band surgery. But I can assure you I felt no pain during, and was actually not just pain-free but quite giddy after it was over.

I remember thinking, back then: *If I wasn't a flight attendant I'm afraid drugs could be an option.*

Now the waiting room at the hospital was quiet, and smelled like stale cheese. I remember looking out of the big glass window all the way down to the parking lot below, picturing my body falling through the air, hitting the pavement. It felt that much like I was in a freefall. When I get nervous I tend to crack jokes to whoever's in earshot. Unfortunately, the woman who checked me in, sitting perched behind a small computer desk at the entrance of the surgery waiting room, had absolutely no sense of humor. My attempts at humor did not even begin to make her crack a smile.

So I reminded myself to grab hold of her at the last moment, if I did decide to leap, and take her along – making the world a happier place.

"Victoria Ashton?"

Suddenly, there she was. The nurse in the green scrubs, just like on "Grey's Anatomy." Except this was not a young, cute actress; more like Rosanne Barr in hospital garb. She smiled at me as I made my way toward her, and that melted some of the icy fear that had layered my skin until it felt like plastic wrap.

Finally, it was time. When I got to the hospital and was weighed in, it turned out I'd lost seven pounds during my week of fasting. YES! I'd heard of people losing even more – but hell, I'd take it. I was no match for those so-called 'perfect' fasters. Hmm, I began to wonder. Perfect, or just not honest? It's fantastic, amazing, a huge accomplishment simply to make it through fast week without cheating. But I sure as heck didn't belong in their category.

And let 'em tell you right now, it was very cathartic to write this down: I weighed two hundred and forty three pounds. *Two hundred and forty three.* I weighed a whole freakin' two hundred and forty three pounds! I, Victoria Ashton, a person who used to take so much pride in her looks. One who used to laugh and dance and sing, and swore she'd never be fat, now weighed two hundred and forty three pounds! Well, by check-in time, two hundred and thirty six.

Yes, that number was hard to take in, at the time. The reality was of it was rough. But I'm ready for this, I told myself. I'll do whatever it takes. Because I am stronger than I ever gave myself credit for – before.

The nurse led me back to a little corner of what looked like an emergency room area, then put me in a smaller room labeled with the number 14.

"You need to take all your clothes off, and put everything in this bag." She handed me a stark white shopping bag which had been standing on the floor at stiff attention. It was like the ghost of a Macy's bag with its sturdy handle, just waiting to be stuffed with great sale merchandise.

"Now, take this sponge and rub the iodine all over your midsection for fifteen minutes," the nurse continued. She did everything but salute and click her heels as she snapped my curved shower curtain shut, leaving me alone with a big bottle of weird orange liquid and my over-hanging stomach peeking out from the hospital prom-gown.

I never knew fifteen minutes could last so long. While I rubbed and rubbed that iodine all over my mid-section, I actually missed her.

By the time she returned, I'd already managed to tuck myself into the bed-on-wheels that took up most of my tiny room. I could see the white top-sheet ripple as a shudder , a manifestation of that fear-of-the-unknown anticipation left my body.

She peeked through the other side of the curtain and smiled in at me. "All set, hon?" she asked. "Oh – do you want me to go get your parents from the waiting room?"

Well, that did it. That was all it took for my breath, which I hadn't realized until that moment I'd been holding, to escape my lungs and push out my clenched lips. I was trying to hold back spasms of giggles, but almost started crying when Jody and Rick entered the room, magazines in hand, unconcealed worry on their faces.

"Hi Mom and Dad," I blurted out, relieved to still be able to laugh, and to appreciate each beautiful face in turn. Needless to say, neither one was amused by my nurse's assumption.

The next thing I knew, in what seemed like only seconds, the anesthesiologist breezed in and started messing with a machine to the left of my bed. "I'll have you knocked out in a minute," he said.

"What?" I gasped. "You'll have me knocked up in a minute?"

His exasperated face did not register any appreciation of my humor, either. Then suddenly, out of nowhere, Dr. Fontana appeared. He pressed cold hands on my orange-dyed belly, and along with encouraging words about my one-week weight loss of seven pounds, put my mind at ease.

People were surrounding the bed by then. I heard the murmured words, "Your first today, Doctor" as a clear face mask hugged my mouth and nose, quietly urging me toward a clear, fluid sleep. Wheels all set in motion, the room suddenly spinning – and I was gone.

Chapter 11: Too Much Love

Two hours after lap-band surgery, I sat on a padded easy chair in the recovery room looking over at my bed, wishing I could just lie down and go to sleep. The nurse had reassured me (in fact, demanded) that I sit up for awhile to avoid clotting or any fluid collecting in my lungs. My twelve-year-old daughter lay across my bed, DS in hand, iPod buds in her ears, and such obvious relief on her face to find her mom was still alive.

My mother and my sister Marina sat chatting on the other end of the bed. My husband and my nine-year-old son had already filled my lap with presents and cards. My two best friends, Jody and Joe, were also keeping a watchful eye on me, though somehow they kept fading in and out of focus. Then my sister Valerie, after traveling all night on a red-eye flight to come see me, raced in and kissed my cheek.

Yes, the room was full of love and excitement, and I was overwhelmed to be the center of all this positive attention. But really, at that postoperative moment, all I wanted of these wonderful, supportive people was for them to get the hell out of the room and just let me lie down.

Finally my wish came true. I slept on and off while Jody, the only one of the gang left, curled up in the easy chair, staking out her spot for the long night ahead.

If I lay still I felt no pain at all. But I'd been instructed to move. So I walked the corridors slowly and carefully, towing the IV bag and pole along like a liquid lifeline. Smiling at my neighbors, totally relating to their weary faces and tired, drooping bodies. Finally, after finding a comfortable position in the mechanical bed, I fell into a deep sleep.

At two o'clock in the morning I awoke with a fever. Jody called for the nurse. My friend's expression worried me as I looked into her frightened, concerned face. The nurse came in and pressed the breath machine into my hands. "Blow hard," she said.

After about thirty minutes, Jody pressed for a doctor to be called, but was dutifully ignored. I looked at her, needing reassurance. Instead, oddly, I felt chilled by a steady calm.

"Breathe," was all the nurse said, pointing to my yellow "breathalyzer" machine, until she was satisfied I was manipulating it correctly. I blew hard, pushing for the little ball to go the full way to its goal, up and down, up and down.

"You need to get up and walk," my mean Nurse Ratchet said.

Man, moving around was the last thing I felt like doing. My stomach was sore. I had chills, too. But I got up and walked for about ten minutes. Thirty minutes later, she took my temperature and I no longer had a fever! Jody and I looked at each other in amazement. Walking and blowing! No more fever! It was like the medical Twilight Zone. I loved that nurse.

The next morning, Dr. Fontana came in and said he was pleased with my progress.

"I'd love to stay another night," I said, certain I'd get more rest in the hospital than at home with the kids, husband, cats, dog, guinea pigs...

"We like for our lap-band patients to go home as soon as possible," he told me. "There's always more risk of infection staying in a hospital than in being at home."

Well, that was enough information for me. By noon, I was up, dressed, saying my farewells to my nursing angels, and ready to hit the road. My husband was coming to take me home. And I was glad to leave, thinking of what Doctor Fontana had said about all the germs present in a hospital.

Still, it was painful to use the energy required to sit up in the car. I was looking forward to lying in my comfortable bed at home. I remember thinking how smoothly everything had gone, how blessed I was. Rick, with a slight whistle under his breath, (which usually means he is feeling anxious) turned onto the freeway, toward home. Smooth sailing... we got it now...home James...

Then, suddenly: ga-lump, ga-lump, ga-lump.

You have got to be kidding me. We looked at each other as we realized what the sound meant. A flat tire! It was like my combination pelvic exam and fire drill all over again. But I tell you, I've never seen anyone move as fast as he did. We were back on the road less than ten minutes later. My hero!

At home, my family was fantastic. I felt like a princess being waited on hand and foot. But by the second day I was going stir crazy. And I was also phenomenally hungry; really craving a steak and salad. In fact, after a while I could not think of anything but steak and salad.

Unfortunately for my gastronomical fantasies, it's recommended that new lap-band patients stick with a liquid diet the first seven days, so swelling around the band site will go down. "You can gradually add soft foods by the second week," I'd been told.

But by day three I was in tears. Absolutely, positively starving.

"Why don't you chew on a steak, then spit it out before swallowing?" Joe recommended. His ex-wife had been through gastric bypass years before. He was passing along her tricks and even some useful bad habits.

Well, I gotta tell ya, it worked. My husband made me a steak and I chewed and sucked it dry, then spit it out. Now this is one more thing I'm not proud of – and I vowed never to do it again and make it some kind of scary habit. That was the only time I ever did that. But that little trick did an amazing job of taking the edge off of my indescribable craving. So I was able to continue with what my bariatric bible told me to do.

    By the end of week one, I was dressed and on my way to a lap-band support group meeting, a list of questions in hand.

Chapter 12: Fourteen and Counting

Lap-band support meetings are held once a month, and at my first one the room was filled with patients in different stages of the treatment. A handful of regulars who'd already had the surgery were religiously there, ready and willing to share their experiences and show off their progress to the roomful of newbie hopefuls. Many there were going through the process I'd just completed. Attending the meeting for information and as a necessary part of completing their must-do, must-have list before surgery can be approved and delivered. Then there were the ones curious about lap-band and attending to just listen in.

I was a little late that evening; the meeting had already begun. A doctor from Norfolk Surgical Group was already up front and speaking as I slithered into a seat in the middle of the room, wincing at the slight tug and pull from my stitches.

"How many of you have already had the surgery, and what were the dates?" he asked.

A handful of people, myself included, raised their hands.

"I had my surgery one week ago on March 12th," I answered, feeling proud at the impressed response that rippled around the room.

"This is a perfect example of what I was talking about just now," the doctor continued. "Many people return to work around three days after surgery."

Whoa. Three days? Now, I don't think I could've done that; not with my job as a flight attendant. For example, after the surgery you're not supposed to lift anything that weighs over 15 pounds, for five weeks. Forget that on a flight! However, with an office job? Possibly I could've made it in to sit at a desk seven days after surgery. But right now, at just one week out, I was still pretty sore. I felt exhausted just from making the ten-mile haul to this meeting.

One woman spoke of being back to work on Monday, her surgery having been done the Friday before. I was truly grateful then for my twenty-nine year seniority with the airline, which allowed me to take six weeks recovery time.

I'd lost fourteen pounds since starting my fast the week before surgery. I seemed to be doing well with different types of food. Mashed potatoes, cream soups, and yogurts all went down well. The problem was, I could not get satisfied and feel really full. I was still hungry–a lot. At the end of my week,

I'd started eating chicken salad with crackers and that seemed to fill me up. But then two hours would pass and I'd want more. This really concerned me. Wasn't I supposed to feel full now?

I raised my hand and bluntly asked the doctor, "Why am I still hungry all the time?"

"This feeling is not rare, and does happen in some cases," he said. "We don't like to give a fill (the saline injection into the lap-band's port to tighten the band) until at least six weeks after surgery. Once you've had that, you should easily feel satisfied."

Many people I've met at lap-band support groups told me they didn't have much pain after the procedure. Well, OK. Great. But I did. Maybe I'm a wimp, but I did feel pain. I talked to one woman who said she never took the liquid pain medicine provided after the surgery. Let me tell ya, I did! Whenever it said I could take some, I did. And it definitely helped. I stayed in bed when I first got home for about five days. Granted, I got up and walked around, but then was happy to make it back to bed when I was finished with that little bit of exercise.

I'm sure it made a difference that I had my husband and children spoiling me and waiting on me hand and foot. I really didn't have to get up and do a lot of things for myself. It was awesome. There they were, cooking for me, fluffing my pillows, encouraging me, loving me. Amazing how I ended up with a man like Rick. Maybe that was a little bit of the reason why I stayed in bed so long... ya think?

I cannot tell you how proud I was of myself to be sitting there in that first meeting. Fourteen pounds thinner, and ready to talk to and try to help anyone who had doubts and needed some encouragement. At that meeting, thanks to asking the question about being hungry so often, I'd found out that you could not have your first fill until six weeks after your surgery. It seems you need to make sure your port site is healed before the doctor puts a needle in it. But I was very anxious to get that first fill. I was feeling so very hungry, so often. And not eating much, of course.

I remember an older man at the meeting who was proudly telling the story of his amazing weight loss. He said, "I haven't had a potato chip since my surgery over a year ago, not since that night."

For some reason that single line, of all the stories told that night, affected me the most. He was so proud of himself, and really wanted to please his doctor. I understood that feeling. We all did. But as he said it, I suddenly had an overwhelming feeling of Food Doom, similar to the one I'd had way back during my Drive-in Fast Food Binge Attack. Oh My God. Was I ever really going to be able to eat again? Specifically, things I really enjoyed. Were pasta and potatoes a total goner now?

I went home and had one potato chip.

Chapter 13: Hit Me with Your Best Shot

After six weeks had gone by, I sat in Dr. Fontana's office feeling a little nervous about our first encounter after my surgery. The last time I'd seen him, I was flat on my back in a hospital bed. I knew I was going to ask for a fill, because the hunger and food cravings were still taking a toll on my psyche. I'm sure my frustration was evident.

Before I saw the doctor, a staff member came in to interview me about my progress. "You've lost fourteen pounds Victoria. That's great!"

"It is?" I replied. "I thought I might've lost more by now."

"One to two pounds a week is what we like to see," she answered, "and you're doing very well. Are you taking Prilosec and your vitamins every day?"

"Yes," I made a sour face. "I'll be happy when I won't have to crush them anymore, though."

"Well it's important to do that until you're completely healed and the pills won't get stuck. How's your hunger?"

"It's there," I replied grimly.

"Are you getting sixty grams of protein a day?"

"You know, I'm not having a problem eating anything. Not eating as much as I used to, but that's because I don't want to gain back the pounds I've lost. I'm kinda freaking out about it."

She reassured me one more time, then left me alone while I waited for Dr. Fontana. I felt tears welling up. *I will not cry, I will not cry...*

"Victoria." Dr. Fontana entered the room, hand outstretched to take my shaking one.

I jumped up and gave him a big hug. Funny how the emotion I put into seeing my doctor, one man who's been an important part of my journey, could make or break my feelings. It felt like longing for the approval of a parent, or a desire to please a favorite teacher. I really hoped to make him proud. And I was so nervous about doing something wrong, because I felt no different yet inside than I had before the surgery.

By then, though, I defiantly felt that food was my enemy.

After looking over my results and my charts, he reiterated everything the nurse had said. "You need to be patient. You really are doing well, right on schedule. Let's give you a fill and see how that goes."

Lying down on the table, revealing my still-sore stomach, I watched as Dr. Fontana checked my incisions and felt around for the port at the end of my band. The stick of the three-inch needle was not as bad as I'd anticipated. Not as bad as a shot; closer to what it feels like to give blood. It was the *thought* of what was taking place that disturbed me. My head and my stomach did give a little spin, but I was also excited about finally feeling what this band was supposed to do.

"Now sit up," he said. "I'm going to give you some water to drink."

You have got to be kidding me. Sit up, with a needle still sticking out of my stomach? OH MY GOD! OH MY GOD! OH MY....

Oh. Okay. Not so bad.

I drank slowly from the paper cup of water he offered.

"Feel that going through?" he asked.

"Nope."

He added another half cc of saline through the needle.

I took another sip. "Nope." I added, "Nothin'."

After adding 2 cc's more he pulled the needle out. I did not feel that at all.

"I'm not going to put in any more right now. Don't eat anything until tomorrow. When you do, eat slowly and chew thoroughly."

I left his office feeling excited, trying to stay confident. I was determined to do everything he said, to make this thing work.

The next day while running family errands I stopped at Taco Bell and got an order of refried beans. Slowly, carefully, I chewed and swallowed while parked in a space in the restaurant lot. I gradually got a feeling of heaviness in my stomach. Halfway through that small cardboard cup of mashed beans, I felt full. Definitely there was a huge difference after getting that saline fill. I went through the rest of my day elated, buying healthy foods at the grocery store, determined to cook healthier for my family.

My children, who had at least once a week craved Burger King, had been suddenly introduced to more vegetables and fruits than ever before in their young lives. Their father was right on board. He also wished to lose the extra pounds his middle had taken on over the last few years. Suddenly, weight was melting from my body. My lost self started to emerge.

Still, I have to admit there were some cravings I couldn't – or perhaps I should say, wouldn't – control. But I was learning how to better manage them. I'm not a big sweets eater (thank God). Give me salt, anything with salt, and I'm happy! Now suddenly, especially at night, I was craving sweets. So I bought my favorite candy, almond M & M's, and on the nights I was going sweets-crazy would eat three of them. Just three. It totally helped my cravings and I was satisfied with just a few of those candies, which I greedily hid from my children. My Diet Pepsi cravings were gone, replaced by a new addiction: unsweetened iced tea with a little Sweet & Low stirred in.

I did try my old habit, experimentally, and found I could tolerate the carbonation. But now my old friend Diet Pepsi tasted too sweet and "tinny." I started to crave – yes, crave – foods like fresh vegetables. Red onions, especially. I cooked lots of chicken stir-fries and ate lots of salads. When I did long for something else, though, I would eat it. I filled up fast, so as soon as I felt that "full" feeling I stopped. I was done.

No longer thinking, living, and dreaming only food. I felt terrific!

Around this time my airline company issued new uniforms. They gave all the employees a budget to purchase new wardrobes. I was unsure of what size to order by then; my last uniform had been a 20. So I ordered pieces in 18, 16 and 14, assuming that would be safe. My big, medium and I-can't-wait uniforms. By then I'd lost twenty-three pounds and my size 18 pants fit great. I didn't feel like a stuffed sausage! When I undressed at night, I no longer had a horrible indentation wrapped around my middle like a huge red ligature mark. That deep, ugly, red-and-raw line which cried out to breathe all day under my tight-fitting clothes.

I started bringing my own food to work – not an easy feat when you go on a four-day trip. If I didn't have my own good stuff along, I ate plenty of salads. After searching, I found that to be one of the few healthy items sold in airport terminals.

***

Six months after surgery I commuted home after a long trip and arrived around dinner time. As I unpacked my son Dylan sat on the end of my bed, watching. "Mom, can we go out to eat tonight?"

"We'll see," I replied. "I was actually looking forward to cooking for all of us tonight. Something healthy." I looked up to see his cute face suddenly all scrunched up, and tears starting to flow. "Dylan? Dylan, what's wrong honey?"

"I'm so sick of eating healthy!" he wailed.

Well, maybe I had been a bit dictatorial with my new-found health regime. Off to Burger King we went for a well deserved special treat for my young hero. And quite a treat it was for me to listen to him order the chicken sandwich instead of his old double-cheeseburger standby. Kaitlin still favored chicken nuggets, but this time opted for mandarin oranges instead of fries! It seemed I was getting through to my children's French-fry-saturated minds. This was turning out to be one of the best years I'd had in a very, very long time.

Chapter 14: The Last Straw

Cocky and confident, I strolled into the little conference room in the hospital I'd come to know so well. I slid into my double-expanded seat, feeling great excitement and anticipation about this meeting. It'd been two months since my surgery, and this follow-up was required for all the hospital's post-op patients. A wellness meeting; an appearance to let the staff know how well or not-so-well we were all doing.

I set my large unsweetened tea down on the large round table and took a long pull from the straw. Michelle, the exercise therapist, took center seat among the eight other women. "Good to see you all today," she said. "If everyone is signed in, let's go around the room and find out how you're all doing."

The first woman sounded positive. She was ten pounds thinner and finding her old energy again.

She was having some trouble eating meat, and so substituting, for her 23grams of protein, the recommended protein drinks for people with this problem.

The next woman spoke of how she'd gone hiking with her family, a thing she had not been able to do in years. Her face flushed with pride as she spoke of her all newest accomplishments.

Then it was my turn.

"Well," I started, "I am twenty pounds less than I was two months ago." Everyone smiled their approval. "And I'm proud to say I jumped on the trampoline with my children for the first time ever."

Granted, I'd only lasted seven minutes, and couldn't walk the next day just from using all those leg and butt muscles I'd thought were nonexistent. But the beaming smile on my boy's face, and my girl's laughter, were enough to carry me happily limping through the week.

"The joy my children were exuding was enough to keep me on a permanent high," I went on. "I'm doing great on the food level. I fill up fast and stop when I'm full. If I go too long without food, I do get a slight burning hunger that Taco Bell refried beans seem to cure." I paused for breath. "I do have a question, though. Why is it we're not supposed to put straws in our drinks? I use them all the time with no problem at all. And I have no problem drinking a carbonated drink as long as I'm not eating at the same time."

Clearly, judging by the faintly-annoyed look on Michelle's face, this was not something she wanted to hear. I sensed real irritation pushing out of her well-toned body, aimed right at my overly-confident chakra.

"Don't listen to Victoria, folks," she said, frowning. "The swallowed air from the straw can cause you real discomfort. And carbonation is not recommended, not only because of the trapped gas it could cause, but also because bubbles could make the band expand. Fran will be here in a minute. She can explain further."

I'd found Michelle a bit intimidating, but Fran definitely had one up on her in that department. She, as our nutritionist, was strict and adamant about food choices, and about following rules. I was not about to challenge her.

When Fran entered, everyone looked over at me as a loud BLUUURP sound filled the small room. That had been me pulling the straw from my fast-food cup and ditching it under the table. Hands now folded like a convent-school girl's on the tabletop, I turned my full attention to Fran, while everyone giggled under their breath.

The next woman in the group to talk was someone I'd seen before. She'd been very heavy then, and to be honest did not look any lighter than that last time I'd seen her. I remembered she had lots of problems besides weight-gain. She was diabetic and had high blood pressure, too. I recalled her talking about all the medications she was on, and about being unsure of how to deal with that when she had to do her seven- day fast.

She told us, "Right after my surgery I was kept in the hospital for four days." Once back home she'd had horrible problems with her diet; frustrated because she couldn't keep any solid food down and kept throwing it up.

Everyone got very quiet as she spoke. We could all feel her pain as she explained that she now felt this surgery had been a huge mistake – for her.

Fran handled it well, though. She assured the woman that help was available to her twenty-four hours a day. And as I looked around I realized that, out of the eight women around that table, there was only one who was unhappy and having complications.

I left that day feeling lucky; blessed that I was doing so well. I swore I'd never take any of it for granted.

***

There is a really cool screening test; one you're not required to do, but something I would highly recommend. It's called the white-light scan. Your first one should be done before the surgery. Then you can get another every three to six months afterward. Let me tell you about it. You go into this little room with a booth, which you stand inside. You're left there alone, so you can go in naked or with underwear on. No one sees you.

You draw the curtain and suddenly are in a black box. You stand with feet apart, both hands gripping bars at your sides. When you're ready, and holding very still, the room goes pitch black and classical music filters in through speakers located around the tiny room. Many, many little beams of light start to dance and twinkle to the music. These beams are actually taking measurements on every part of your body. After about twenty seconds you're done. Painless!

   The computer technician on the other side of the curtain then steps out so you again can have privacy and get dressed. Then she shows you a lovely, computerized image of your body in all its glory. You don't see precise details but, believe me, the overall effect is stunning. I looked at my stomach – or should I say, stomachs. One lovely roll on top of the other. Yuck. My upper thighs were smushed together, my breasts looked like two watermelons and my butt... well let's just say I inherited that flat heart-shaped rear end my mother always proudly wiggled around. And still does, might I add.

   In just a couple days you receive your light scan results in the mail. It was amazing and horrifying at the same time to see all those measurements. I had my second scan done three months after surgery, and it was quite uplifting to see the progress; such a significant difference with all of the crazy inches I had lost. I no longer had three chins! Everyone I knew had started to make comments about the weight loss there.

   "I can see it in your face."
   "Your face looks so much thinner."

I saw a big difference, too. My face now sported a huge smile; one that had not been seen for a very long time.

Chapter 15: Bad Breath Heaven

What was also amazing is the foods I continued to crave after the surgery. The new, pleasant reality was that I - a former junk food aficionado - now longed for vegetables. Especially, as I mentioned before, red onions. I know, go figure. At one point I wanted a red onion so badly I could've eaten it like a crunchy Red Delicious apple. On my next visit to Dr. Fontana I asked sheepishly, "What vitamin's missing, that I need onions so much? What does that mean?

"Well," he answered, as I waited with the breath pulled deep into my lungs, expecting some secret lack of an obscure mineral. "I believe it means...that you like red onions."

Yowza. But it's true. Even now I really do feel like I have to eat them at least once a day. My family doesn't love it, though, since my kisses always are smelly.

Then, for some reason, bell peppers came into play. The orange, red, and yellow peppers in salads and stir-fries colorfully calling to me to gobble them up. Stir-fry with chicken or pork, the peppers, and onions (of course), along with fresh green beans, asparagus, broccoli, almonds, snap peas, snow peas, bok choy and bean sprouts. All are now a constant in my kitchen. The leftovers are fabulous, and a mugful at lunch time fills me up and makes me smile at the same time. Honestly, as the weight began to melt, potato skins and nachos dropped from my food vocabulary. Yeah! I'm not kidding. I don't know why, but sure am not questioning it. I have also felt extremely proud and happy to see my kids really take to healthier choices as well. Not all veggies are a hit with them, but we've learned they love broccoli and zucchini. To me, that's a wonderful start.

Now I don't stock the kitchen cabinets with chips, cookies and candy like I used to, because what's not there can't be tempting or get devoured. Instead I buy a ready-made veggie platter with low-cal ranch dressing and put it out on the kitchen table just before they get home from school. After some time on the backyard trampoline or just running around with Issy, our dog, in the back yard, those veggies are gobbled up and appreciated. Cucumbers with a little salt sprinkled on fill the kids up too, and refresh them for hours.

One thing I am very grateful for is that my children love water. They did not get this wonderful trait from me or their father, considering we were both Diet Pepsi freaks. So I always make sure our garage fridge is well-stocked with bottled water.

Once in a while on an airplane ride, or in a restaurant, they'll order a Sprite or some juice, but in the end it's usually wasted. Yet bottles of water disappear left and right in our house! Thank goodness for little miracles.

Now, me? Mmmhf. A whole different story. I still do not like plain old water. I'm sure I must've downed at least a six-pack of Diet Pepsi the day before my surgery, though. Yet now I was doing fine without sodas since, as Michelle the exercise therapist nurse noted, the carbonation at times could feel uncomfortable. I did pick up a replacement addiction: unsweetened ice tea with Sweet & Low. A pitcher of that has become a permanent fixture in our fridge, since my husband also gave up his soda habit. I also love Crystal Light or any of the sugar-free powders that can be used to flavor your water. We definitely have been saving some money by not purchasing crates and crates of diet sodas, as in the old days.

People seem to think that eating healthy and buying good-quality fresh foods is a lot more expensive than opting for the old prepackaged junk. That they wouldn't be able to afford to regularly eat things like lean meats, fresh cheeses, and beautiful fresh fruits. Well guess what? Yes, you can. I added up a week of fast-food eating, Hamburger Helper meals, boxed macaroni and cheese, miscellaneous junk food, and already-prepared meals versus the healthy way I cook now with fresh vegetables and lean meats. I discovered I save money by preparing it all myself – because you can make more, freeze some for the following week, and make your food budget actually go further.

For Christmas I received from Santa three amazing little booklets entitled *Eat This, Not That*. One is for comparing healthier grocery store foods with pre-packaged and frozen foods. Another is all about the real ingredients in fast foods, and which are the healthier options if you must choose to eat at one of these places. The third booklet was written for children, and with great excitement I introduced to my kids. We were all flabbergasted to learn some of the foods you think are healthy are actually full of preservatives, salt, and sugars. Even fast-food salads! For instance, a yogurt parfait from one place actually has thirty grams of fat in it!

These books were really good for my kids to read. Now they understand what they are actually putting in their mouths. I see them looking and thinking before they make a decision about what to eat. OK, not always . . . but hey, even most of the time works for me. For instance, my daughter and I went to lunch with some friends recently, and she ordered a turkey wrap without mayo instead of her favorite fried-chicken fingers with French fries dipped in ranch dressing.

While we were eating she turned to me and said, "Thanks, Mom. I really feel better when I eat this way. But I wouldn't be doing it if I didn't see you always trying so hard."

My heart soared. Then a few minutes later she told me she was still hungry, and ordered a side of fries. Sigh. Little steps.

Still, after you read the grocery guide from *Eat This, Not That,* you cannot help but let it guide you to better choices at the store. It's really interesting how subconsciously knowledge affects us.

For instance, I recently visited my sister in Ohio and went grocery shopping for us when I got there. She was floored at the choices I'd made when she helped me unpack all the brown paper bags.

"Wow Victoria, I've never seen you shop this way."

"Yep." I nodded. "If someone else is having something I really miss, I'll treat myself to a bite. But usually, if I take the time to stop and think of a food choice I'm making, I will be satisfied after eating only that much . . . and more important, guilt free!"

Well, guess what? I am never going back to the way I used to shop. Ever!

Chapter 16: Your Tool

By August my weight loss seemed to be happening pretty fast. In six months I hit the two-hundred mark on the scale, and then could not wait to get below it! It'd been years since I'd weighed less than that. The sole exception was when I was on the Atkins Diet and went below two hundred for all of about two minutes.

Every morning I looked at the scale with great anticipation, just waiting for that sacred moment. Two hundred, two hundred and one, two hundred and three, two hundred, two hundred and two. Ugh! I stayed on a plateau just like that for about two weeks. Then one morning, out of a clear blue sky, the scale said one hundred and ninety eight. I did it! I'd gotten below that damn two hundred mark. Happy dance!

Getting there involved some struggle and discipline. There are important rules you're supposed to follow in order to have success with the lap-band. For example, you're only supposed to eat three small meals a day. You must... and listen, I mean must, eat slowly. Chew your food very thoroughly. Believe me, I know. This was one area where old habits would come into play, and I'd suddenly, conveniently get very forgetful. Feeling hungry, I'd simply gulp down a couple bites of something without thinking. Old habits do die hard.

Each time I did this, instantly I knew I could be in trouble. So right away I'd take a couple of gulps of water, then get rid of the problem food I'd swallowed by literally just coughing it up, before it had a chance to go down and possibly get stuck. I know...eww. It's not pleasant to contemplate. But far better, believe me, than having a wad of food get stuck, and then being in pain for two days.

In the lap-band world, a big key to success really is to stop eating when you feel full. And let me tell you... that can happen pretty quickly. All this means is that your smaller stomach is full, and you should not still be hungry even if you stop after a few bites. If you feel full, you are full.

Another important tip: Do not drink liquids while eating. If you're chewing and grinding food properly it will pass through your band into your larger stomach slowly, without a problem, and without needing liquids to move it along.

Also, do not eat in between meals. You know what? I don't have a problem with that one. At least, not now! I'm never hungry between meals any more. Actually I only eat lunch and dinner, which is quite common, according to Dr. Fontana. Most of his patients only eat two meals a day after lap-band surgery.

Now I will admit there are times where I feel hungry late at night. I know, I know-you're not supposed to watch television while curled up in bed before going to sleep, but I stand guilty as charged on this point. It's the way I unwind from my work day. Unfortunately I tend to get the munchies while doing so. But I've made a great discovery for salt addicts: pumpkin seeds in the shell. I suck on a seed, bite it like a pistachio nut, discard the shell and eat the inside. I end up eating only a small handful, and they are quite satisfying.

Next tactic? Try to eat only quality meals. Well, yah. That's not rocket science, I know. And yes, I'm eating healthier than ever before in my life. Occasionally I'll even treat myself to a soft-serve ice cream cone from Dairy Queen. But the key is just that... on a special occasion.

Next one up is to try to avoid fibrous foods. They can get stuck in the band and cause discomfort, or even severe pain. More on what happened when I disregarded this warning, in an upcoming chapter.

Do make sure to drink plenty of fluids during the day, when you're not eating. This practice makes a huge difference and it keeps you hydrated. Very important! In fact, it's a must. But do drink only low-calorie liquids. Otherwise you can quickly sabotage and stop weight loss, or even gain additional weight by drinking milkshakes, sugary sodas, any sugar-added drinks, sweet fruit juices, or alcohol. These are all choices that simply spell excess, useless calories.

Now for the big tip: EXERCISE. Unfortunately this is a hard one for me. But if I can do it, believe me, so can you! The trick is to find a fun way to get fit. Then I know I can and will stick with it.

Dr. Fontana, and my brain... they both insist on exercise. But a bit of serendipity also didn't hurt. After I'd lost about thirty pounds, I went into a liquor store to purchase some margarita mix for a cook-out we were planning to have over the weekend. In the store sat a beautiful cream-colored beach cruiser bicycle, part of a giveaway sponsored by Malibu Rum, and they were raffling this bike off. So I put my name in with the hundreds of other entries already there, took my margarita mix and left.

"I want a beach cruiser bike," I dropped on my husband when I got home. "I could really get into riding up and down the boardwalk by the ocean."

That weekend we went shopping and looked at the beach cruisers in bike shops. But I could not justify shelling out three hundred dollars for a whim, even a seemingly healthy one. So I let the thought go. I'm happy to shell out for a special fun camp for my kids, or new clothes for them, or piano, guitar, dance lessons, ya-da, ya-da. But a bike just for me? No way.

Well, a month and a half later, while at work on a Chicago overnight, I got a phone call. "Is this Victoria Ashton?"

"Yes," I said suspiciously, not recognizing the number on the cell phone screen.

"This is ABC liquor store. Congratulations! You won our beach cruiser!"

Get out of town! I never win anything. And from a liquor store, of all places! Clearly the God of Workouts was looking out for me. I guess someone had to – because Dr. Fontana, I can still hear your words: "Victoria, you must exercise."

Right. And away I go.

Chapter 17: All Hands on Deck

One thing that's very helpful to the lap-band's success is getting the rest of the family involved in making meals. My son has taken to it very well. He's loved to cook since the age of two. This past month he was featured in our local newspaper as the 'Everyday Chef.' Dylan has a lot of talent for preparing food and has made it his hobby. He loves to eat, too. He and I have been learning different recipes, though, since I had my surgery. If I take extra time to prepare his meals, rather than just slapping a greasy bag filled with cholesterol and fat in his hands, it not only makes him feel better, it makes me feel like a good mom. These are our children, people. We need to say no to fast food places, just as we do to drugs. To teach them one of the most important lessons of their young lives: How to eat to live in a healthy, happy way. Not simply to live to eat.

I still am learning how to eat out in restaurants, though. Some of that experience has been a bit of a trial. The doctor will give you a medical card explaining that you are a bariatric patient, asking that you be allowed to order a kid's meal because a full-size order is just impossible to finish. And unless you can take your portion home and eat it for the next couple of days, you're going to get way too much food, and then have to waste what's left.

But there's another really big problem. Have you looked at what they're serving for children's restaurant meals nowadays? Fried chicken fingers, corndogs, cheeseburgers, pizza, spaghetti and fries, fries and more fries. This is why I let my kids order off the main menu, as long as it's a better choice than that kid-meal crap.

I've found just two restaurants so far that offer kids' meals which seem any good. We eat there often, all ordering the kids' portions, which are plenty of food for all of us. Ruby Tuesday's has a wonderful grilled chicken breast served with broccoli and mashed potatoes. You can include a salad from the abundant bar for a little extra. But watch out for the tons of calories in some salad dressings. Every choice counts! Max and Erma's has the same children's meal. Many times I so get a full-size order (they will prepare it any way you ask) and take the rest home. That will last me for usually two more lunches.

I also have had margarita cravings, which of course I limit. But I gotta tell ya, I crack Doctor Fontana up when I tell him I've got no problem eating the chips and salsa. Now I can't eat a lot, but I can definitely eat it. I can handle corn tortillas of any kind without a problem, but I cannot eat the ones made from flour. They're just like eating glue, to me. You know, those served with fajitas? One of my favorite things to order in a Mexican restaurant has always been the fajitas. I love to eat the sizzling meats and veggies right off the hot platter. But no flour shell. And usually, unless I've shared, I take some home. The next day I'll put a corn tortilla in the microwave, on a paper towel, for ten seconds. Then roll up the leftovers in that. Yummy!

I've also been using my grill... a lot. I have no problem with proteins grilled to perfection, along with (of course) grilled red onion and other wonderful veggies. My friend Joe and I have perfected the baked potato. Put it in the microwave until soft, about ten to fifteen minutes. The big secret: brush the potato with oil, then salt it. Put on the grill for a crispy wonderful outside and fluffy bliss on the inside.

***

Another area I've tried to incorporate and change is the lunches my kids take to school. The norm used to be a ham or turkey sandwich with mayo and lettuce, a bag of chips, some cookies and a whole apple or orange. This lonely fruit pretty much always made its way back home in their lunch bags every day.

Then I heard through the grapevine that my daughter didn't like sandwiches and usually gave hers away or traded for something else. It turned out I'd been feeding someone else's child for years! So I started to try new, more creative lunches. I found a way to preview them by making first as an after-school snack. Kaitlin loves peanut butter, and Jif (her favorite) even makes it in these handy little individual servings. I started to pack a serving of peanut butter and some fresh celery or carrots in place of a sandwich to dig into it. She loves it! Or I cut up an apple and let her dip and scoop the peanut butter with the apple pieces.

She also loves BBQ potato chips. Lays has come up with a baked chip you can also buy in the small lunch-bag size. Any flavor of Yoplait yogurt is a great dessert. So is one of those 100-calorie cookie packs, which are just big enough to satisfy that sweet tooth. Now don't get me wrong, every once in a while I throw in Dad's homemade cookies, or some store-bought insanely-chocolaty-chippie cookie. But she claims to be really into my healthy lunches now.

My son loves hot food. So I went to Target and bought him an awesome camping thermos which costs a little more than the standard plastic school thermos, but it is so worth it because it keeps the meal so hot. Now, instead of something canned like Spaghetti-Os, I give him a chicken, broccoli and pasta lean cuisine, or shrimp linguine. He loves them; all the varieties. He's developed a bountiful food palette, and is not a picky eater like his sister and Mom.

For desserts at home they eat Smart Ones key lime pie or brownies. I also love to serve fresh strawberries with a big dollop of Cool Whip on top. I'm not a big sweets-eater but that hits the spot with me, too. I feel just as good about watching my family change their eating habits as I do about me changing mine and losing weight.

***

My family used to really watch me in the beginning while I ate. If I made any kind of face, or even set my fork down, they'd say, "Is it stuck? Are you okay?" Now they're used to my slow, precise eating and know I'm just fine. I still adore food, but I eat much, much less. I'm starting to like my body again. Forty eight years old and rediscovering myself. Who knew?

Now I can really, honestly say, "Do as I do." It makes everything come together, you know? Making the whole surgery experience even more worth it.

Chapter 18: And Now: What Not To Do

I was one month away from my surgery's one-year-anniversary date when I received my second fill. Afterward, Doctor Fontana warned me about not eating anything for at least twenty four hours. He also knew I'd be off on a work trip for a few days. "Don't eat until tomorrow, Victoria. You need to give it time. Especially since you're going out of town."

Damn, it was exactly two p.m. The time I always just start to get hungry, I thought. And now I can't eat until this time tomorrow? Why didn't I eat something before I came in for this darned fill! Now I'll be starving by sundown.

Sure enough, in the hotel that night my stomach kept growling. I was thinking only about food. I couldn't concentrate on anything, including sleep. By chance I had some Triscuits in my bag; my favorite cracker – before surgery. I'd still occasionally chew on one; a forever task, now. But this night, without too much thought, I ate three in a row, pretty fast. Not chewing a million times, which would've undoubtedly made a difference.

About ten minutes later I could feel the crackers were stuck in my band. As was my habit, I drank some water and tried to throw the blockage up. I tried so hard that my chest soon felt on fire but the scratchy crackers stayed put. It was definitely painful. I drank more water hoping to dilute them and help them pass. Still nothing but pain. Dry heaves and pain. I sat on the floor in that old hotel bathroom in Philadelphia with my arms wrapped around the toilet bowl, and cried. Why hadn't I listened to Dr. Fontana? After two hours I finally fell into a restless sleep.

The next day, while contemplating whether to call in sick for my trip and go home, I drank a couple of deep sips of water. Like a small blessing, I suddenly threw up the crackers. What emerged looked like an inch-long cork plug, along with some blood. Which, I gotta tell ya, freaked me out. The pain immediately stopped, but I'd already started to imagine all types of bad things going on in my body. *I bet I messed up my band. I tore something in my stomach and there'll be this big emergency, and I'm away from home and... and...and.*

I picked up the phone and called Dr. Fontana's office. With tears clogging my voice I confessed my sins to his nurse, Barb.

"Why did you eat those crackers?" she scolded. "You shouldn't have eaten them."

Well, yah, I think I already had that part figured out.

"You just really irritated the site where the band is," she announced. "Eat puréed food, soft stuff like soups for a couple days. Stay away from anything scratchy or rough like Triscuits."

Ta-da! You're kidding, right? No problem. NEVER again. No more Triscuits for this girl. Soups, mashed potatoes here I come. And two days later, I was as good as new. I absolutely love Barb.

***

My friend Jody now lives in Ohio, but I couldn't wait for her to witness my progress. I jumped on an airplane and went for a weekend visit.

Her reaction was not exactly what I'd expected. She looked me up and down, then pouted. "I want lap-band surgery."

Jody has struggled with her own weight, but never gotten to the point where I'd been. Nor does she have any of the health issues I'd been battling for so long. It's important to know that the lap-band is not a quick and easy fix simply for weight gain. It is a specific tool. One that only works it if you work it. (Where have I heard that before?) You cannot get the surgery just because you are overweight. You get it to save and to improve your life, and you must need it for medical reasons. You must be ready, and you must take responsibility. From the outside it might look like an easy fix. But the truth is, I still must work at maintaining my weight and making the right food choices every day. To date I've lost seventy pounds, and am working towards losing fifteen more. But honestly, if I just stayed at the weight I am now, and healthily maintained it, I'd be okay with that. My energy level, my outlook, everything is so much better in my life, it just makes me smile and smile.

***

One thing I had worried about was scarring. I've always scarred very easily. But I gotta tell ya, I have a worse scar from where I once had a mole removed, than the scar from my lap-band surgery. The most obvious mark is the one-inch scar left from when Doctor Fontana placed the port. It's just a tiny line, not even raised. The other places that marked where the surgeon made incisions are now gone. The staff did warn me that if you expose the scars to sunlight, they can get worse. I use a tanning booth every so often, (okay, okay not that often!) and I always make sure my scar is covered up. But really, it doesn't look bad at all.

I was also worried about sagging skin, after the fat was gone. Especially on my belly, because that's where I carried the most weight. But lo and behold, I'm okay. I'm not saying I don't need some toning; I definitely do. But for the first time in years I actually think I look okay in a bra and underwear. I don't think I would wear a bikini on the beach! I feel too old to go that far, now. Although, I don't know... Valerie Bertinelli is my age and, va-voom, she looks good. Her own weight-loss is definitely an incentive for doing some push-ups and toning, now that much of the flab is gone.

Hers has been an interesting story for me to watch. When I heard Valerie's interview I zeroed in and related to so many of her past frustrations. She did not have as much to lose as I did. But let's face it, any weight is hard weight to lose. I tried Jenny Craig... twice. And Nutra-System. And Phen-Phen. And Alli.

Jenny Craig's food was good. I would start out well for the first couple of weeks. But eventually the dinners I was cooking for my family would start to look too good to resist. One bite led to two. Two bites would lead to "I'll just eat with them tonight. Tomorrow I'll start again." Wrong! I did like the accountability factor, but the frequently-rotating staff at the Jenny Craig Center did frustrate me. Every time I'd think I was going in to see someone familiar at the end of the week, a person I'd been bonding with and getting used to, there'd be someone new. It was like starting fresh, all over again.

I'm sure there's a lot of motivation to lose weight when you're doing it publicly, but it seemed like Valerie really plugged in and made it work. Me? Afraid I'm more like Kirstie Ally. Once you're not watching me, BAM. I'm a goner.

Weight Watchers was another dilemma for me. I'm a lifetime member, so does that tell you how many times I've gone to them? It is a fabulous program if you follow it and practice it correctly. At one time, when I was weighing in at one hundred and sixty five pounds, (I'm 5'7 and a half) my then-boyfriend told me I was too fat for him. Wonder who that was? Yep, good old Andrew. I went to Weight Watchers so he could see a written account of my weight loss, and basically starved myself. I got down to one hundred and twenty-five pounds. If you'd seen me then, I looked not just skinny but anemic. He liked me that way, though, so of course I wanted to please him. I remember crying myself to sleep at night wondering what would happen if I put even a morsel of food in my mouth. Yes, I know: I was sick, and in an even sicker relationship. He didn't care how I did it, he just wanted me thin. I ultimately decided I would rather be alone forever, rather than have a relationship with someone like him again.

I truly believe most of the relationships in my past contributed to my weight gain. I always got involved trying to find some self-worth. I was never alone, but nice guys always finished last as I went on my conquest for chaos. The abusive ones, in one way or another, were usually those I stayed with for any length of time.

I built some very important and meaningful relationships with friends at that time, though. This is the period I met Jody, and she and I had similar pasts. I was very into the arts. Anything creative, and I was there. Acting and love of theater introduced me to a handful of gay men who never let me down. I could totally be myself around them. I never felt judged, and yet there was also really nothing I could get away with. They knew me inside and out. All my friends wanted to protect me from life, but what I really needed was protection from myself. I was still the one saying to me, "You're too fat, you're too thin, you're not happy enough, you're not smart enough, you're not enough, not enough, not enough. ENOUGH!

The rare instances I was without a boyfriend were probably my best of times. I connected with family, and spent more time with friends, and just let myself be. Those were the best of times and yet-because I still hadn't learned how to like and take care of myself – those were the worst of times, too.

Chapter 19: Another Scary Evening

I had my third fill in November. Everything went well, and I felt fine. I was eating less and less by then. After I was given a little over two CC's with the fill, I could really tell a difference in how much food I could eat. But by January I started experiencing pain in my back every time I had a meal. Both sides of my lower ribs was where the ache came from. I started asking whoever I was eating with to rub those spots on my back, and that seemed to help.

Yet as the days went on, after I ate the pain would at times become unbearable. Then I noticed even liquids were not passing through my band easily, and realized I was not getting enough fluids. Yet, selfishly – and really not thinking too brightly – I let this situation continue. Because, of course, I was seeing such a rewarding amount of weight loss.

Meanwhile, everyone close to me was saying, "Call Dr. Fontana."

"Oh, I have a follow-up appointment in twenty-three days," I'd answer, frustrated with all the concern. The truth is, I really knew something was wrong, and was scared to see him.

Finally in February, while out on a work trip, I experienced the worst pain yet in my back, right after eating lunch. I knew then I could not put off calling the doctor. It would hurt for hours until the food passed and then I would feel fine. But this process was exhausting and after a while I didn't want to eat, for fear of the pain.

He worked me in immediately after my return and decided to x-ray the band while I drank another glass of that lovely, chalky white liquid. (Honestly, they really need to invent something that tastes good for those procedures.) Despite my worries, it was actually kinda cool. I stood, and the machine was behind me, but the picture appeared on a monitor n front of me. He had me drink the nasty stuff. We watched it travel down to my small pouch of a stomach-and then stop. Just stop. No draining through to the larger stomach at all. It didn't go down, up, out, or anywhere.

Dr. Fontana did not seem very pleased. "Victoria, how long have you been living with it like this?"

Actually, I didn't know. I'd simply accepted the pain, and tried to just ignore it. I liked the fast weight loss too much. Bad decision! He put a needle in my port and drained my band of all of its fluid. Instantly I felt relief as I watched the liquid that had been stuck drain through to my lower stomach.

"There is nothing really wrong," he told me. "Just too much fluid in the band. It made the opening too tight for anything to pass through. But," he stressed, "you need to tell me if you ever feel any pain. There's no reason to live like that, and no reason for you to be in pain."

I hung my head, feeling as if Yoda was shaking his finger at me. Sniff.

He replaced some of the fluid in the band with the needle, while I drank water and we watched so not too much was added. Boy, did I learn my lesson. I have not felt any pain since. I will never, ever allow myself to feel that way again. The band is not supposed to hurt people! Remember that. If anything does hurt or feel uncomfortable, you need to go see your doctor ASAP! Don't be stupid like I was and live with unnecessary pain. Stupid . . . when my goal is to act as smart as I know I am!

Chapter 20: Loose is Out

Many lap-band patients, including me, have trouble holding food down in the morning, or whatever time they eat the first meal of the day. It's important to remember the opening to your larger stomach is now only about the size of a dime. Drinking some liquids before you attempt food is a good idea. Three or four times, while making breakfast for my kids before school, I've been tempted by a piece of turkey bacon, or to take a bite of bagel. This has never worked. Each time I had to immediately drink some liquid so I could go and throw up those stuck impulse-bites.

Eventually, you do learn. In the beginning I'd find myself popping something into my mouth unconsciously. Then, luckily, thinking: What the heck am I doing, and spitting it out. I think half the things I ate while fat must've been swallowed without thinking, too. I didn't even realize I was putting them into my mouth.

When I shop for clothes now I still tend to pick those larger "non-stick" shirts and lug them to the dressing room, only to be surprised when they hang loose and limp off my shoulders, like I'm merely a hanger from my closet. Now that clothes fit, I actually enjoy shopping for them.

People who've know me a long time react to the new Victoria in different ways. Some seem uncomfortable, seeing such a big change. They have a hard time looking in my eyes when we meet. Others come right out and gasp, "Wow, you've lost a ton of weight!"

I actually prefer the latter reaction. My persistence this past year at working with my lap-band tool, and becoming openly honest about weight and health issues makes me want to be noticed and admired. It was not an easy task. Now I want to share it with the world.

***

My third white light scan was amazing. I made my appointment and could hardly wait to step into that little black box. I'd just seen Dr. Fontana and gotten the great news that my BMI was now at 26. Holy cow. At seventy pounds lighter I felt as though I was walking on air. Music, lights, action, I smiled and stood as still as possible so the beams would take an accurate measurement of my body.

When I stepped out the nurse showed me my image on the computer. "It looks really good Victoria," she said.

I frowned and looked at myself more critically.

"Hey girl," she said. "Look at the Before. Then look at the After image. This one looks really, really great. You can't get much better than this."

Ahhhh, but yes grasshopper, I can. And I will.

***

I love sales. I've been having fun buying groceries, because it really is possible to save with coupons and still eat healthy, wonderful foods. The newspapers have amazing sales. Many times Joe and I used to go to the store when they had Buy One, Get One Free specials, and then split the cost. That's just too cool. The biggest thing I learned was to not go grocery shopping when you're hungry. I've been teaching my kids how to read labels and to understand brand versus store names. Now they both get a kick out of receiving a good bargain.

I've lost weight in increments so keeping clothes that fit rather than sagging off me can be hard. But who am I to complain? I finally took it upon myself to clean out my closet and get rid of all my old fat-clothes. I did go shopping after the first forty-pound weight loss and spent at least seven hundred dollars. Yet none of those clothes fit me now. So I've discovered secondhand shops and in casing them have found some incredible bargains. Being a flight attendant I'm blessed to be able to pick up nice overnights. Although we do have great consignment shops where I live, I've found some fabulous ones on my Los Angeles overnight. Never-used, unbelievable clothes and shoes. For forty bucks I got a pair of leather pumps, a leather jacket, French boots, and a really cute top. Brand-spanking new. Love it! Who wouldn't love to shop for bargains, especially since they fit so well now? Thanks to the lap-band, my hard work, and a growing awareness that exercise plays a vital part in keeping this new me fit and happy.

***

The first time I'd felt like exercising was that day I jumped on the trampoline with my son. For seven whole minutes! I think I only lasted that long because his face was lighting up the sky. The next day, thanks to those seven heavenly minutes, I could not walk. I came down the stairs one slow step at a time, at each one saying Ouch. Oh my gosh. Oww. Everyone laughed at me, but muscles were aching that I didn't even know I still had.

A couple days later I decided to take our golden retriever Isabel for a walk. Now she was not in the best of shape either, even though she took jaunts around the backyard every day. All in all, Issy was a lazy old dog. I snapped the leash on her collar. With my son at my heels saying "Mom, I want to go, I want to go" – off we went.

I lost them both after the first mile. Issy went from dragging me along to a slow, sloppy walk, to her wet nose poking at my heels.

"When are we going to make it home?" Dylan whined as he dragged to keep up. I tell you, if I'd had my cell phone along, I would've called Rick to come pick up both my slackers.

A car passed slowly through the neighborhood, and Dylan started to wave it down.

"What are you doing?" I yelled.

"Maybe he'll give us a ride, Mom," he said.

Oh my gosh. Had all my warnings and words been wasted on small, deaf ears? "Dylan," I scolded. "You never, never get in a car with a stranger! You never, never . . ." Blah, blah, blah.

He just stared at me through tired little eyes. Fifteen minutes later we trudged through the front door. Isabel drank a gallon of water, and Dylan passed out on the sofa. We've all got to get in shape I thought. Wow.

That night I spoke with my husband about my fears of having a lazy family. Our kids were not overweight, but I was going to do all I could so they wouldn't have to go through, and more important, feel what I've felt about my own body, as an adult.

My son now plays baseball (so far their team is undefeated. Go Dodgers!) My daughter dances, and got cast in the musical "Grease" with our local theater group. We are all water babies, and plan to swim a lot this summer. I've become obsessed with watching the Food Channel. You can really pick up some healthy ways of cooking there. Extra virgin olive oil and garlic are now our staples for many healthy meals.

I still don't always make the healthiest choices. But when you read and educate yourself about what's not healthy you tend to pass by many things in the grocery store. I want my children to learn how to cook well. It's just too easy to stop and purchase an already-made, but usually unhealthy meal. We used to go to Subway and Dylan would order meat, meat, meat sandwiches. Pepperoni, salami, ham, turkey, beef, extra cheese, mayo, wow. Now I tell him we will only go to Subway if he thinks before he orders. He stands at the counter, his ten-year-old brain actually clicking, and then orders turkey, with cheese, lettuce, pickles and light mayo on whole wheat bread. He gets a pack of baked Lays potato chips on the side, and a big, big water.

My daughter Kaitlin orders the same way. I love to watch them thinking about their options and ordering from their brains, not their stomachs. Yes, I have influenced them. And, most importantly, empowered them with knowledge. But if I let them take the time and think about it they come up with those choices themselves. I really try to cook as much as I can when I'm at home. Many nights I'm tired; many nights it feels hard. Ordering a pizza would be so much easier! But I just keep picturing my old self in my head, and the path I want for my family, and that makes it much easier. There is no better feeling than the knowledge that you are giving your family the chance for a long, healthy, productive life.

***

Remember the bike I won? This past holiday weekend my best friend Joe and his daughter invited the four of us to go bike riding on the trails of Seashore State Park. Okay, I admit it. I've been living here in Virginia Beach forever and have never ridden a bike on those trails. I'm not a big nature person, although I do love the ocean. Not swimming in it, mind you, but I do love the sight of the ocean. When I was younger I loved to ride my bike down the ocean boardwalk, bikini top and shorts on, soaking up the sun, traveling that nice, even pavement. Stopping at Raven Cafe for chicken wings and beer, then moseying back up onto the boardwalk. But among the trees? With bugs and snakes?

My kids got excited about the outing, though, and my husband was happy we were going to do a family thing. So I like the good mother I am, I packed up a great picnic lunch in a really cool basket Joe and I had found on one of our yard-sale treasure hunts. We put all the bikes into the van or on racks, then off we went.

Riding the first half-mile of trail was okay, even though it was far from a nice, smooth boardwalk. Tree roots jutted out, small rocks were flying all over the place, and we had to dodge under low tree branches and around sand pits. That was not fun. If anyone was to say, "Let's think of a way to make Victoria miserable", this ride would rank in the top three best ways.

The kids and Joe raced ahead. Rick, with his butt off-balance from the heavy picnic basket attached to the back of his bike, and me with my eyes riveted to the ground, picking gnats and mosquitoes from my teeth, lagged behind. Then, lo and behold, I spotted a beautiful patch of color ahead; a lovely shade of mango. I smiled at the pretty color until the mango-spot moved, or rather slithered across the trail about a foot in front of my bike. Black body, mango stomach, 50,000 feet long, I swear. While I didn't scream, I sure speeded up.

After about five miles we stopped for lunch at a beautiful lake right next to the trail. Lunch, of course, was the best part. We always enjoy each other's company and my food was pretty good – and healthy. Then, not two minutes after hitting the trail again, another – or maybe the same one, who knows – black-mango snake undulated across the path in front of me. This time I almost ran over it. This time I did scream! "Okay, I'm done. Where's the parking lot?"

Five miles later my son let out a shout as if he'd just seen a ghost. I raced to his side. There on the trail in front of him lay another fine, skinny black friend, this one with a whitish belly. We watched it slither away as I calmed Dylan and myself down. After what seemed a long, hilly lifetime later, we made it back to our cars. As I sat red-faced n the front seat, listening to my son proclaim what a good time that had been. I turned the cool air on full force.

When my husband got into the van he looked over at me sheepishly. "I'm proud of you," he said. "You did really good."

"Don't talk to me," was all I could squeak out.

The next day I told my mother that story and had her rolling in fits of laughter. "You must be so sore!" she said.

That's when I noticed. If I could've just put the bitching aside for one moment, I might've realized I wasn't really sore. That I actually felt great. No pains, no aches. Even my butt wasn't aching from that darned bike seat. A year earlier I could not have made that trail ride for one single mile without getting red-faced, sweaty, and out of breath! Yet I'd just pedaled ten miles and the next I didn't feel sore! What a revelation. Hallelujah!

Chapter 21: Looking Back; A Checklist from My Former Life

When I was a younger flight attendant, as I mentioned before, we used to have to get weighed by the company once a year. If we were overweight we wouldn't be allowed to fly. When I graduated from training I was nineteen years old and weighed one hundred and thirty five pounds. Seven years later I stood on my supervisor's scale and watched as the dial showed us an unfamiliar number: One hundred and fifty.

"Victoria," she said. "You really need to get your weight down."

I was not at the mark where I wouldn't be allowed to fly, but close.

As the years went by, eventually the airline stopped weighing us. We have no weight restriction now. In recurrent training, which we go through every year, they check your fitness (and weight) by seeing how fast you're able to fit through exit windows. Still, I cannot tell you how many times I wished we'd kept that demeaning weigh-in ritual. Maybe then I wouldn't have allowed myself to get to a whopping two hundred and forty three pounds.

Two hundred and forty three! That number doesn't even seem real to me now.

My family has always talked about weight, though. My mother and my two sisters and I could not spend time together without weight somehow or another becoming an issue. It's still that way today. My sister Valerie and I have always been the worst yo-yo dieters. She can relate to my weight struggles the most. She, too, can go up and go down. If I went up in weight, it seemed she was going down - or vice-versa. Right now, thank goodness, we are both down. I cannot count how many vacations we took together with our children, saying, "We're going to be good all week. We're only going to eat healthy." Once, we went to Sanibel Island and decided to try the Atkins Diet together. It was going pretty well. We were religiously eating our cheese, bacon, egg, steak. Meat, meat, meat. After about four days on this diet we took our kids to an ice cream shop on the island. While they were picking out what flavor their cones were to be, Valerie and I looked up at the television screen in the corner. It was blaring the news that Dr. Atkins had dropped dead on a New York street. Shocked, we just stared at each other. Then, we both got ice cream.

I know Mom was sad when I got fat. She didn't really comment too much on it. I think she knew I was sad about it, too. Sometimes she'd try to help, in her way. Like signing me up for a Curves membership, or suggesting we go to Weight Watchers together. But this sort of outside offer only made me sink lower into depression. I know now I was simply not ready to unbelt the layers of protection that surrounded my body. For years I'd had very low self-esteem: not smart enough, not pretty enough, not confident. Yet people who saw the surface thought I was all those things, while those who knew my soul constantly, consistently told me I had to learn how to love myself.

I can honestly say that, this time, after lap band surgery, I actually am for the first time starting to feel a real, positive, connection to myself. Not just because I'm finally doing what's good for me. And not just because I'm still continuing to lose weight. But because I feel like I am worthy of losing it, at last.

I first wrote these words at writing retreat in Sedona. I could see and feel the birth of this book coming through my fingers. My thirteen-year-old daughter texted from her cell phone, telling me to stay positive: MOM IM SO PROUD OF YOU. Out of the mouths of babes!

My mother, in her mid-60s when my father died, was left with countless bills. She was devastated when she had to sell her home. Yet I've watched her blossom into the strong, confident woman she is today. She never gave up. It's never too late to go looking for yourself. It's never too late to learn, to grow.

The message I want to end with is this: Don't be afraid to ask your doctor if lap- band surgery could be right for you. Take the time to research all there is to know. Make sure you ask all the questions are on your mind. Most importantly, if you are not comfortable in any medical situation, then change it. It is very important to have the right medical team beside you. They become like family; they guide you and work by your side for success. To date I've lost seventy-two pounds. My life has changed drastically. I hope my story has been an inspiration to you. And with that, I bid you good luck, good life – and get goin'!

THE END

Victoria's List: My Old Nightmare Existence

1. Airplane seats got tight
2. Jump-seat seatbelts cut into me
3. Double, triple chin
4. Thighs rub together when walking
5. Out of breath just walking up a flight of stairs
6. Sweating, sweating, sweating
7. Hot flashes all the time
8. No male attention from strangers
9. No female attention from strangers
10. Walking by a mirror and seeing my own reflection
11. Baggy clothes. T-shirts, T-shirts and more T-shirts
12. Tight uniforms cutting into my stomach
13. Tired all the time
14. Hungry all the time
15. Sad all the time
16. No endurance, no stamina to play with my children
17. Buying huge bras
18. Buying old lady panties
19. No pretty nightgowns
20. Uncomfortable to wear high heels

21. Bumping into things because I didn't realize how big I was
22. People saying "You have such a pretty face."
23. My 86-year-old mother had more energy than I did
24. Sleeping a lot, then wanting to sleep more
25. No self-esteem
26. No ambition
27. No willpower
28. Feeling lazy and unmotivated
29. Feeling old
30. Feeling that time is running out.

Glossary of Terms

Anesthesia: The loss of sensation and feeling. Also refers to the process or drugs used to produce this effect. Anesthesia is commonly employed prior to surgery so that a patient will not feel any pain or discomfort.

Bariatric: Related to the branch of medicine that deals with the prevention and treatment of obesity.

Bariatric Surgeon: A surgeon who specializes in the surgical treatment of obesity.

Body Mass Index: The most widely-used measurement for obesity. The BMI approximates body mass using a mathematical ratio of weight and height (weight in kg divided by height in meters) or (weight in pounds divided by height in inches times 704.5). A BMI of 30 or more is regarded by most health agencies as the threshold for obesity. A BMI of 40 or more generally qualifies as morbid obesity. However, BMI measurements in body-builders and athletes may not be accurate determiners of obesity because the BMI does not distinguish between muscle and fat.

Comorbidity: A medical condition that exists along with, and is caused or worsened by, obesity or any other primary disease being studied or treated. With sufficient weight loss, obesity-related comorbidities such as Type-2 diabetes, hypertension and sleep apnea generally improve or may be completely resolved.

Diabetes Type 2: A chronic endocrine disorder characterized by the body's inability to properly utilize sugar, specifically glucose, a simple carbohydrate. This results in excessively high glucose levels in the blood. Diabetes means there is either a relative or an absolute shortage of insulin, a hormone that regulates the body's breakdown of carbohydrates. A higher percentage of obese individuals have Type-2 diabetes than does the general population.

Dumping Syndrome: A physiological reaction frequently seen following gastric-bypass surgery, an operation designed to alter the function of the stomach and intestines, to deliberately interrupt normal digestion. Thereafter, whenever patients eat certain foods, such as sugar and sweets, they may experience "dumping," characterized by symptoms of nausea, flushing and sweating, lightheadedness, and watery diarrhea. This complication has been reported by most gastric bypass patients. Lap Band patients do not suffer from it.

Gastric Bypass: A surgical procedure for the treatment of obesity where a thumb-sized stomach pouch is created using stapling techniques to divide the stomach and then connect the outlet of the pouch directly to the intestine (also called the bowel), essentially "bypassing" the lower stomach. The flow of digestive juices is preserved, however. This procedure achieves its effect by restricting the volume of food consumed and also the type of food that may be consumed. Sugars and fats can cause "dumping syndrome." Gastric bypass surgery can be performed via open surgery (one large incision) or less invasively with laparoscopic techniques (several tiny incisions), although laparoscopic gastric bypass is performed infrequently. Produces rapid and significant weight loss, but is associated with higher mortality and complication rates. Also known as Roux-en-Y or RNY.

Gastroesophageal Reflux: The backward flow of stomach contents into the esophagus due to a malfunction in the sphincter at the end of esophagus. Reflux can cause heartburn and discomfort. When it occurs repeatedly, it may become gastroesophageal reflux disease (GERD), where stomach acid eventually causes scarring of the esophagus and other chronic problems.

Heart Disease: Any number of diseases related to the heart and blood vessels; also known as coronary artery disease. When grouped together, these diseases are the leading cause of death in the United States.

Hypertension: The medical term for high blood pressure. Usually, this means that a patient has blood pressure of 140/90 or higher. For older adults, this number is adjusted upwards slightly. The top number is systolic pressure (pressure in blood vessels when heart is pumping out blood), while the bottom number represents diastolic pressure (when heart is at rest). This condition is also associated with obesity, due to the excess weight the heart must sustain.

Ideal Weight: Generally, this term refers to what a person of a given height and body frame should weigh; in other words, the desired weight for optimal health and fitness. There are several problems, however, with currant calculations of ideal weight: a) body fat percentage or distribution is not accounted for; b) only some of the tables account for different body frames or ages; and c) most importantly, there is no medical consensus about which formula or table to use. Thus, ideal weight remains subjective. To illustrate the variation, a height of 5'6" plus a medium body frame for a female has an ideal weight between 124 and 149 pounds, depending on the source.

Laparoscopic Surgery: A minimally invasive surgical approach in which the surgeon makes several small incisions to access the interior of the body. A long, slender camera, attached to a light source, and chopstick-like instruments are used to perform the operation. Compared to the large incisions used in conventional open surgery, there is typically less pain and scarring following this operation. Usually, hospital stay and overall recovery time are also reduced.

Laparoscopic Gastric Bypass: A minimally invasive method of performing gastric bypass surgery. The surgical risks, however, are comparable to that of standard gastric bypass. It is used infrequently, though, due to the difficulty and complexity of the procedure.

Morbid Obesity: A disease in which excess weight begins to interfere with basic physiological functions such as breathing and walking. Generally, it can be defined as weighing at least 100 pounds more than your ideal weight. A more precise indicator, however, is a Body Mass Index (BMI) of 40 or greater. In addition, a BMI of 35-39.9 with significant comorbidities can qualify.

Obesity: A condition in which there is excess body weight due to an abnormal accumulation of fat. Defined objectively as a Body Mass Index (BMI) of 30 or more, obesity is associated with markedly-increased health risks.

Sleep Apnea: The temporary cessation of breathing during sleep. Typically, the sufferer will awake gasping for breath. Sleep apnea may occur repeatedly, resulting in a poor night's sleep and daytime drowsiness. One of the comorbidities also associated with morbid obesity.

Stoma: The outlet to the stomach created by stapling or placing an adjustable band around its upper part, which divides the stomach into two parts: the smaller upper stomach pouch and the lower stomach. This results in restriction of the amount of food the stomach can hold and increases the time it takes to digest and empty. The Lap-Band allows the stoma to be adjusted when a doctor inflates or deflates the inner surface of the band in order to modify the degree of restriction.

Stroke: A sudden loss of brain function due to a blockage or rupture in a blood vessel that supplies oxygen to the brain. Depending on which area of the brain is affected, a stroke may lead to muscular coordination problems, slurred speech, blindness, paresis (weakness), unconsciousness, paralysis, coma or death. One of the comorbidities associated with morbid obesity.

ACKNOWLEDGMENTS

Here's where I say thanks to everyone who made this book possible. Lenore Hart: for believing my story was worth telling; without her I would not have had the courage to write the truth. Rick : for insisting I was smart, and teaching me in color. Kaitlin and Dylan: my children. My soul. Loving their mom through her fat, thin, cranky, happy, up and down days! Jody and Joe: by my side, in my heart. Valerie, Marina, Sharon: relating to the pain and reveling in the joy. My doctor, Mark Fontana. My writing Guru, Tom Bird; photographer, Robert Ander; and my publisher, Northampton House Press. Thank you, thank you, thank you! And finally my mother, Nina. In this journey as her daughter, I have learned strength, determination, and devotion to not only the ones who love me, but to myself as well.

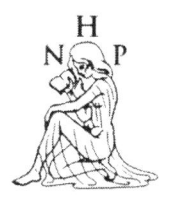

Northampton House Press

Northampton House LLC publishes carefully selected fiction, lifestyle nonfiction, memoir, and poetry. Our logo represents the muse Polyhymnia. Our mission is to discover great new writers and give them a chance to springboard into fame. We try to publish books that offer something new to the marketplace, and to readers; works that have up until now been overlooked by large trade houses. Our watchword is quality, not quantity. Watch the Northampton House list at www.northampton-house.com, or Like us on Facebook – "Northampton House Press" – to discover more innovative works from brilliant new writers.

Made in the USA
Charleston, SC
07 March 2013